COMPLICATIONS

T   es

World Health Organization
Geneva
1995

WHO Library Cataloguing in Publication Data

Complications of abortion : technical and managerial guidelines for
   prevention and treatment.

   1. Abortion – complications 2. Abortion – prevention & control 3. Maternal
   mortality

ISBN 92 4 154469 4   (NLM Classification: WQ 225)

The World Health Organization welcomes requests for permission to
reproduce or translate its publications, in part or in full. Applications and
enquiries should be addressed to the Office of Publications, World Health
Organization, Geneva, Switzerland, which will be glad to provide the latest
information on any changes made to the text, plans for new editions, and
reprints and translations already available.

The designations employed and the presentation of the material in this
publication do not imply the expression of any opinion whatsoever on the part
of the Secretariat of the World Health Organization concerning the legal
status of any country, territory, city or area or of its authorities, or concerning
the delimitation of its frontiers or boundaries.

The mention of specific companies or of certain manufacturers' products does
not imply that they are endorsed or recommended by the World Health
Organization in preference to others of a similar nature that are not
mentioned. Errors and omissions excepted, the names of proprietary products
are distinguished by initial capital letters.

TYPESET IN INDIA
PRINTED IN ENGLAND
93/9774—Macmillan/Clays—7000

CONTENTS

Contents

Contents

PREFACE

In 1967, the World Health Assembly in resolution WHA20.41 recognized that abortion constituted an important health problem for women in many countries. The consequences of unsafely performed abortion account for a large share of maternal mortality and those who survive may suffer long-term sequelae including infertility.

National authorities are responsible for deciding whether and under what circumstances to provide services for the medical termination of pregnancy. WHO takes no position on the matter. However, it subscribes to the view, as recommended at the International Conference on Better Health for Women and Children through Family Planning, Nairobi, October 1987, that, "Regardless of the legal status, humane treatment of septic and incomplete abortion and post-abortion contraceptive advice and services should be made available."

As noted in the principles of the World Population Plan of Action, reaffirmed and expanded at the International Conference on Population in Mexico City in 1984, the medical termination of pregnancy is not considered by WHO to be a family planning method. However, the level of induced abortion or of abortion-related mortality is a clear indication of unmet needs for family planning.

The primary purpose of these guidelines is to contribute to the reduction of maternal morbidity and mortality associated with abortion. The health care systems in all countries need to address the health care needs of women suffering from complications of abortion. Furthermore, induced abortion, as and where allowed by law, should meet minimum standards of safety and quality.

The guidelines have been produced by WHO's Maternal Health and Safe Motherhood Programme, and are addressed primarily to programme managers responsible for the planning, implementation, supervision and evaluation of women's health care. This book is not intended as a clinical text because abundant technical literature exists on clinical issues. References to key technical sources are included in the appropriate chapters.

The term "manager" is broadly applied within these guidelines to refer to members of the health team involved in planning, organizing, administering, delivering and supervising abortion care programmes and services. In many locations, health managers may also be trained clinical service providers. The guidelines should be useful to decision-makers who are responsible for a national health system, to managers who oversee a group of service delivery points, and to the staff of individual health facilities.

The immediate objectives of this publication are:

— to provide managerial guidelines for improving the quality and availability of care for abortion and its complications, as part of a primary health care system;

— to provide guidelines for the prevention of unsafe abortion and its consequences, in view of the significant role that abortion plays in maternal mortality and morbidity;

— to assist national and local managers in the collection and application of information useful in planning the location and content of emergency abortion care at each level of the health care system.

These guidelines were prepared on the basis of a vast review of literature, information gathered during the course of WHO-supported research on health aspects of methods of induced abortion and their service implications, review by many experts and programme managers working in the field, and the recommendations of a scientific working group which undertook an in-depth review of the text.

Every attempt has been made to make these guidelines of practical value for those responsible for establishing and administering maternal and child health services within health care systems. Thus, separate chapters on planning for services, facilities and equipment, cost-effective management, providing information and counselling to patients, training and supervision, and monitoring and evaluation of services are included along with several annexes that provide suggestions and examples of training materials and record forms that can be easily adapted to local needs. These guidelines are meant to be flexible; the aim is to present important issues and make suggestions that can be adapted to the social and cultural circumstances of each country.

It is not the purpose of these guidelines nor is it within the terms of reference or policy of WHO to advocate or propose the modification of any country's legal code with regard to abortion.

Comments and queries on this publication are welcome, and should be addressed to: Maternal Health and Safe Motherhood, World Health Organization, 1211 Geneva 27, Switzerland.

ACKNOWLEDGEMENTS

The World Health Organization gratefully acknowledges the contribution of staff of the International Projects Assistance Services (IPAS) in Carrboro, NC, USA, who assisted in the preparation of these guidelines, in particular, Sallie C. Huber, Ann H. Leonard, Donald Minkler and Judith Winkler.

An outstanding team of international health professionals participated in the working group that produced the final version of these guidelines. The working group participants included: Raymond Belsky, USA; Grace Delano, Nigeria; Robin Hutchinson, Canada; Khama Rogo, Kenya; Pramilla Senanayake, Sri Lanka; and Margot Zimmerman, USA.

The World Health Organization acknowledges the valuable contributions of the following to the preparation and review of the text: Halida Akhter, Daniel Ampofo, Maybelle Arole, Syeda Begum, Mark Belsey, Pouru Bhiwandiwala, Paul Blumenthal, Marc Bygdeman, Meena Cabral, Davy Chikamata, Rebecca Cook, Adrienne Germain, David Grimes, Kelsey Harrison, Jozef Kierski, Suporn Koetsawang, Olayinka Koso-Thomas, Uta Landy, John Lawson, Deborah Maine, Suman Mehta, Laban Mtimavalye, Jane Mutambirwa, Joaquin Nunez, Viveca Odlind, Herbert Peterson, Praema Raghavan-Gilbert, Shan Ratnam, Yan Ren-Ying, Alberto Rizo, Allan Rosenfield, John Ross, Mamdouh Shaaban, Irvin Sivin, Joseph Speidel, Sudha Tewari, Louise Tyrer, Judith Tyson, and Vivian Wong.

The financial support of the Andrew Mellon Foundation towards the preparation and production of these guidelines is gratefully acknowledged.

Chapter 1

INTRODUCTION

Hundreds of pregnant women, alive at sunset last night, never saw
the sunrise this morning. Some died in labour, their pelvic bones too
small and distorted by malnutrition in childhood to allow the free
passage of the infant. Some died on the table of an unskilled
abortionist, trying to terminate an unwanted pregnancy. Others died
in hospitals lacking blood to control their haemorrhage, and others
died in the painful convulsions of eclampsia, too young to bear
children in the first place and never seen for antenatal care. These are
the women of Asia, of Africa, of Latin America—today
(H. Nakajima, Director-General of the World Health Organization,
October 1990).

WHO estimates that throughout the world approximately 500 000
women die every year from pregnancy-related causes. A large
proportion of these deaths are attributable to complications of
abortion. Further, 98% of maternal deaths occur in developing
countries, where a woman's lifetime risk of pregnancy-related
death is compounded by the greater number of pregnancies
experienced by each woman, as well as by socioeconomic
conditions and the limited availability of maternal health services
in these countries (WHO, 1991).

The dramatic disparity in maternal death rates illustrated in
Table 1 suggests that the large majority of these deaths are
preventable. Improving access to adequate health information and
health care, including prevention of unwanted pregnancy, can
play a critical role in reducing these terrible losses.

Maternal mortality and morbidity

No one knows exactly how many women die each year as a result of
becoming pregnant. Most of those who die are poor, they live in
remote areas and their deaths are accorded little importance. In the
parts of the world where maternal mortality is highest, deaths are
rarely recorded and even if they are, the cause of death is usually not
given (Royston & Armstrong, 1989).

A maternal death is defined by WHO as the death of a woman
while pregnant or within 42 days of termination of pregnancy,
irrespective of the duration and the site of the pregnancy, from

Table 1.   Changes in maternal mortality (around 1983 and 1988)[a]

Region	Live births (millions)		Maternal deaths (thousands)		Maternal mortality (per 100 000 live births)	
	1983	1988	1983	1988	1983	1988
World	128.3	137.6	500	509	390	370
Developing countries	110.1	120.3	494	505	450	420
Developed countries	18.2	17.3	6	4	30	26
Africa	23.4	26.7	150	169	640	630
Eastern	7.0	8.8	46	60	660	680
Middle	2.6	3.0	18	21	690	710
Northern	4.8	4.9	24	17	500	360
Southern	1.4	1.3	8	4	570	270
Western	7.6	8.7	54	66	700	760
Asia[a]	73.9	81.2	308	310	420	380
Eastern[a]	21.8	24.6	12	30	55	120
South-eastern	12.4	12.5	52	42	420	340
Southern	35.6	39.6	230	224	650	570
Western	4.1	4.4	14	12	340	280
Latin America	12.6	12.2	34	25	270	200
Caribbean	0.9	0.8	2	2	220	260
Central	3.7	3.5	9	6	240	160
South	8.0	8.0	23	17	290	220
Northern America	4.0	4.0	1	1	12	12
Europe	6.6	6.4	2	1	27	23
Oceania[a]	0.2	0.2	2	1	300	600
USSR	5.2	5.2	3	2	50	45

[a] Figures for Australia, Japan and New Zealand have been excluded from the regional estimates, but are included in the total for developed countries. Numbers of maternal deaths and maternal mortality ratios are World Health Organization estimates. Numbers of births for 1983 are United Nations estimates for 1980–1985 (United Nations, 1982). Numbers of births for 1988 are United Nations estimates for 1985–1990 (United Nations, 1991). The regional figures may not add up exactly to the regional totals owing to rounding errors.

any cause related to or aggravated by the pregnancy or its management, but not from accidental or incidental causes. Wherever and whenever it occurs, the death of a woman during her reproductive years—approximately 15 to 44 years of age—is a tragedy both for her family and for society.

Women in the developing world have a much greater risk of pregnancy-related death than do women in the developed world. In the developed world there are 5–30 maternal deaths per 100 000 live births, but in developing countries the figures range from 50 to 800 or more. Moreover, a woman living in a developing country faces a risk of death up to 250 times greater if she has to seek services from an untrained, unskilled abortionist than if she has access to a skilled provider and hygienic conditions. The risk of death is significantly reduced when women have access to safe legal abortion services. For example, in the United States of America from 1980 to 1985, the death rate associated with abortion was 0.6 per 100 000 procedures (Henshaw & Morrow, 1990).

Although accurate data on maternal mortality are difficult to compile, the magnitude of the problem is such that the absence of exact measures of incidence should not inhibit the design of health policies and programmes to combat this problem (Rosenfield & Maine, 1985).

Reliable data on pregnancy-related morbidity are less available than mortality data. However, one recent analysis suggested that, for every maternal death, approximately 10–15 women suffer pregnancy-related morbidity (Measham & Rochat, 1987). This would suggest that, each year, approximately 5–7.5 million women worldwide suffer non-fatal but frequently debilitating health problems related to pregnancy.

The role of abortion in maternal mortality and morbidity

Induced abortion is the oldest, and probably still the most widely used method of fertility control. Yet because it touches on some of the most profound religious and moral issues, few societies have been able to look dispassionately at the health aspects of abortion as it affects the woman (Royston & Armstrong, 1989).

The tragedy of maternal deaths is that virtually all are preventable with proper management (WHO, 1986). Globally, around 15% of maternal mortality results from unsafe abortion, and the proportion is as high as 50% in some areas. The high level of mortality worldwide that results from unsafe abortion could be prevented by providing ready access to treatment of abortion complications, safe abortion procedures and contraceptive services (Mahler, 1987).

Unsafe abortion, i.e., the termination of pregnancy performed or treated by untrained or unskilled persons, and its complications are a major direct cause of death among women of reproductive age (WHO, 1986). Recent estimates suggest that around 15% of the more than 500 000 pregnancy-related deaths in developing countries each year may result from complications of unsafely induced abortion (WHO, 1993) and some experts put the figure considerably higher (WHO, 1991).

Regardless of whether an abortion is spontaneous or induced, subsequent events and the care received determine whether the abortion is safe or unsafe. Estimates based on death certificates from 24 countries reveal that between 6% and 46% of all reported maternal deaths can be attributed to complications of all types of abortion (Liskin, 1980).

To illustrate the need for safer abortion practices and services, WHO has compiled a database on unsafe abortion. Data from 67 studies in 17 countries, contained in this database, indicate that, in some areas, up to 50% of maternal deaths occurring in hospital are due to complications of unsafely induced abortion. In many countries this proportion averages about one-quarter of all maternal deaths in hospital (Table 2) (WHO, 1991). Most abortion-related studies are hospital-based. In addition to deaths that occur in hospital, an unknown number occur outside institutions. There have been few large prospective or retro-spective community studies on the incidence of abortion, and

Table 2. Percentage of maternal deaths due to induced or septic abortion in hospital-based studies

Region	Country	Period	No. of studies	Percentage of maternal deaths due to abortion[a]
Africa	Ethiopia	1979	1	30
	Ghana	1963–1967	2	4–7
	Kenya	1972–1977	1	22
	Nigeria	1966–1985	5	6–51
	United Republic of Tanzania	1974–1984	4	13–25
	Zambia	1982–1983	1	15
	Zimbabwe	1972–1983	4	18–32
Asia	Bangladesh	1978–1979	6	15–31
	India	1962–1985	17	3–34
	Malaysia	1967–1973	2	23
	Pakistan	1961–1983	4	2–12
	Philippines	1964–1986	2	16–24
	Thailand	1977–1978	1	25
Latin America	Chile	1960–1979	4	26–46
	Colombia	1963–1978	7	23–45
	Jamaica	1971	1	33
	Venezuela	1961–1973	5	20–70

[a] Table includes only studies where abortion was specified as induced or septic. When the type of abortion was not mentioned, the study was not included.

of those that do exist, several of the most extensive were completed some time ago.

Spontaneous abortion, or the unprovoked interruption of pregnancy (also called miscarriage), affects approximately 10–15% of all known or suspected pregnancies. While spontaneous abortion often requires treatment or hospitalization, it is less often fatal than unsafely induced abortion.

Complications of all types of abortion are also a leading cause of morbidity for women in developing countries. Though the incidence is known to be high, accurate data on morbidity related to unsafely induced abortion are often even more difficult to obtain than mortality data. Infertility, chronic disability, transfusion-related infections and emergency care for complications of unsafe abortion are additional challenges to be faced in the quest for safe motherhood.

Worldwide data on mortality and morbidity associated with elective abortion are likewise difficult to determine with accuracy. In countries with reliable health statistics, recent information about elective abortion demonstrates the relative safety of the procedure (Table 3).

Table 3. Number of elective abortions, associated deaths and mortality rates for selected countries[a]

Country (dates)	No. of abortions (thousands)	No. of deaths[b]	Mortality rate (per 100 000 abortions)
Bulgaria (1980, 1984, 1987)	374	5	1.3
Canada (1980–1987)	511	1	0.2
Czechoslovakia (1976–1983)	781	3	0.4
Denmark (1976–1987)	269	2	0.7
England and Wales (1980–1987)	1095	14	1.3
Finland (1976–1985)	154	2	1.3
Hungary (1980–1987)	649	5	0.8
Netherlands (1976–1983)	509	1	0.2
New Zealand (1976–1987)	74	0	0.0
Norway (1976–1987)	70	0	0.0
Scotland (1976–1987)	101	2	2.0
Sweden (1980–1987)	261	1	0.4
United States of America (1980–1985)	9446	54	0.6

[a] The term elective abortion refers only to those performed legally under the sanctions of the particular country.
[b] All data are based on death certificates, except for England and Wales where deaths are recorded on abortion notification forms and United States of America where deaths are associated with abortion only after investigation.

Sources: Henshaw & Morrow, 1990; CDC, 1990.

When restrictions on abortion are lessened, the number of deaths related to induced abortion is reduced, presumably owing to the greater safety of the procedures performed by trained health professionals. For example, in the United States of America, death rates due to abortion fell by 85% in the five years following legalization (Tietze, 1981).

Fig. 1 graphically illustrates the impact of restrictive legislation on deaths due to abortion in Romania. Romania's permissive abortion law was changed to a more restrictive one in 1966 and by 1984 the number of deaths due to abortion increased by 600%. When abortion became legally available once again in January 1990, abortion mortality fell by 67% in the first year (Romanian Ministry of Health, 1991).

It is difficult, if not impossible, to categorize women who will require abortion care. Women of all ages and walks of life experience spontaneous abortion and also use induced abortion to terminate unwanted pregnancies. Older women of higher parity often seek abortion as a means of avoiding additional births; unmarried, nulliparous adolescents undergo abortion in order to

Fig. 1. Effects of the introduction in Romania, in November 1966, of an anti-abortion law, and of repeal as from 1 January 1990

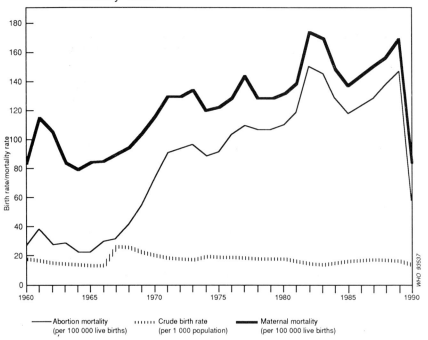

Abortion mortality (per 100 000 live births)　　Crude birth rate (per 1 000 population)　　Maternal mortality (per 100 000 live births)

delay childbearing. Existing statistics indicate that, in most regions of the world, urban dwellers and more educated women are more likely to obtain induced abortion than rural and less educated women. However, this may be only a consequence of greater access to information and wider availability of services or to better data collection in urban areas.

Improving maternal health through high-quality abortion care

While estimates of the incidence of abortion vary widely, it is clear that health care workers are frequently called upon to provide care for women undergoing, or who have undergone, abortion. Any bleeding in pregnancy, whatever the cause, has the potential to cause serious complications and requires emergency assessment and management. These women need emergency care which must be provided even where there are legal restrictions on induced abortion. Assessment of the woman's condition and provision of services must be available on a 24-hours-a-day basis from the point at which the woman first contacts the health care system to the point at which she receives the care she requires. (See Chapters 5–7 for more information on clinical management.)

Reduction of the need for induced abortion and prevention of unsafe abortion through provision of family planning services should be an integral part of health care. Health care providers, women and the community at large must understand the health risks of unsafe abortion and the advantages of contraception as a safer alternative. The incidence of unwanted pregnancy, induced abortion, and related maternal morbidity and mortality can be greatly reduced by increasing the availability of family planning services and providing accurate information to women, health care workers and the community. The full integration of family planning into maternal and child health services is a key component of WHO's strategy for providing improved primary health care for all people.

References

CDC (1990) Abortion surveillance, 1986–1987. *Morbidity and mortality weekly report, CDC surveillance summaries,* **39**: SS-2.

HENSHAW SK, MORROW E (1990) *Induced abortion: a world review, 1990 supplement.* New York, Alan Guttmacher Institute.

LISKIN LS (1980) Complications of abortion in developing countries. *Population reports,* Series F, No. 7.

MAHLER H (1987) The Safe Motherhood Initiative: a call to action. *Lancet,* **1**(8534): 668–670.

MEASHAM AR, ROCHAT RW (1987) *Slowing the stork: better health for women through family planning.* Technical background paper prepared for the International Conference on Better Health for Women and Children Through Family Planning, Nairobi, Kenya, October 1987 (available from the Population Council, Dag Hammarskjold Plaza, New York, NY, USA).

NCHS (1990) *Vital and health statistics—Supplements to the monthly vital statistics report: advance reports, 1987, Series 24: Compilations of Data on Natality, Mortality, Marriage, Divorce and Induced Terminations of Pregnancy, No. 4.* Hyattsville, MD, National Center for Health Statistics.

ROMANIAN MINISTRY OF HEALTH (1991) Directorate for Maternal and Child Health. *Mortalitatea materna.* Bucharest (unpublished document).

ROSENFIELD A, MAINE D (1985) Maternal mortality—a neglected tragedy; where is the M in MCH? *Lancet,* **2**(8446): 83–85.

ROYSTON E, ARMSTRONG S, eds. (1989) *Preventing maternal deaths.* Geneva, World Health Organization.

TIETZE C (1981) *Induced abortion: a world review, 1981,* 4th ed. New York, The Population Council.

TIETZE C, HENSHAW SK (1986) *Induced abortion: a world review,* 6th ed. New York, Alan Guttmacher Institute.

UNITED NATIONS (1982) *United Nations demographic indicators of countries: estimates and projections as assessed in 1980.* New York, United Nations.

UNITED NATIONS (1991) *United Nations demographic indicators of countries: estimates and projections as assessed in 1990.* New York, United Nations.

WHO (1986) Maternal mortality: helping women off the road to death. *WHO chronicle,* **40**(5): 175–183.

WHO (1990) Romania: on the road to success. *Safe motherhood: a newsletter of worldwide activity,* Issue 3: 1–2.

WHO (1991) *Abortion: a tabulation of available data on the frequency and mortality of unsafe abortion.* Geneva (unpublished document WHO/MCH/90.14; available on request from Maternal Health and Safe Motherhood, World Health Organization, 1211 Geneva 27, Switzerland).

WHO (1993) *Abortion: a tabulation of available data,* 2nd ed. Geneva (unpublished document WHO/FHE/MSM/93.13; available on request from Maternal Health and Safe Motherhood, World Health Organization, 1211 Geneva 27, Switzerland).

Chapter 2

OVERVIEW OF ABORTION CARE

Health care services at all levels must be prepared 24 hours a day to provide emergency care for the complications of abortion in line with the personnel and equipment available.

This chapter defines abortion and describes the different categories of abortion care. It also describes the levels of service in typical health care systems and presents recommendations for the components of abortion care that should be available at each level.

Definition

Abortion is the termination of a pregnancy before the fetus is capable of extrauterine life. Further refinements of the term depend on the cause of the abortion. Spontaneous abortions (sometimes called miscarriages) are those in which the termination is not provoked, whereas induced abortions are those caused by deliberate interference. Induced abortions include those performed in accordance with legal sanctions and those performed outside the law. The term therapeutic abortion, strictly defined, refers to medically indicated abortion for women whose life or health is threatened by continuation of pregnancy or when the health of the fetus is threatened by congenital or genetic factors. In common usage, however, therapeutic abortion is often applied to all legally sanctioned abortions. The clinical stages of abortion are outlined in Table 8 on page 42.

Categories of abortion care

The terms emergency abortion care and elective abortion are used throughout these guidelines to describe the two main categories of services.

Emergency abortion care refers to the life-saving services that must be available in every health care system to meet the needs of women suffering complications of abortion. The most common diagnosis for women who arrive at a health facility in need of emergency abortion care is incomplete abortion. Incomplete abortion, if untreated, can lead to haemorrhage, shock, sepsis and death, Treatment includes complete evacuation of the uterus and timely management of other complications.

While emergency abortion care is immediately necessary for preserving the woman's life or health, *elective abortion* is undertaken at the request of the woman or on the recommendation of the woman's doctor. Most legally induced or therapeutic abortions fall into this category. Legal restrictions governing the availability of elective abortion vary greatly and are beyond the scope of this book. Managers should apply these guidelines for abortion care within the legal framework and medical standards of the country in which they work.

Levels of health care

Abortion care should be made available as close to people's homes as possible and should be carried out by the least specialized personnel who are adequately trained to perform it safely and well.

The prevention of abortion-related maternal mortality is dependent on emergency abortion care being integrated throughout the health care system of the country—from the most basic rural health post to the most sophisticated tertiary level facility. At least some components of emergency abortion care— health information and education, stabilization and referral, uterine evacuation, or specialized care for the most severe complications—must be available 24 hours a day at every service delivery site in the health care system.

Although different terms may be used to refer to them, the health care systems in most countries include the following levels:

- the community level
- the primary level
- the first referral level
- the secondary and tertiary levels.

Table 4 lists the type of service facilities available at each level. The following sections of this chapter describe the staff and the elements of abortion care that should be available at each of these levels to provide emergency abortion care. Table 5 summarizes this information.

Table 4.   Service facilities available at
            each level in a typical health
            care system

Level	Service facilities
Community	Community-based health workers
Primary	Nursing posts
	Dispensaries
	First aid stations
	Health posts and centres
First referral	District and cottage hospitals
Secondary	Regional hospitals
Tertiary	University teaching hospitals
	Specialized national hospitals

In some countries, elective abortions are provided in specialized facilities; however, a complete discussion of the management of these facilities is beyond the scope of this book.

Community level

Health care workers at the community level can play a key role in reducing abortion mortality and morbidity, particularly in remote areas far from formal health care facilities. In the villages or hamlets of many countries, health education and basic services are delivered by individuals who operate outside the formal health care system, often working out of their homes or a community building. These individuals—traditional healers, *curanderos*, traditional birth attendants, and other community residents— attend to the basic health needs of the community in which they live.

Village health workers are often the first people contacted by women who have bleeding or pain in pregnancy or who wish to terminate an unwanted pregnancy. In addition, in many areas of the world, traditional health care workers perform unsafe induced abortion. It is extremely important that cultural concepts and beliefs governing the practice of village health workers in handling abortion be understood throughout the referral network of the health system. Community health workers need to be informed about the dangers of unsafe practices and dissuaded from carrying out these procedures. These individuals must be motivated to educate the community about prevention of unwanted pregnancy and encouraged to refer women to the formal health care system promptly when they need treatment that cannot be provided at the community level.

Table 5. Emergency abortion care activities by level of health care facility

Level	Possible staff	Care activities
Community	Community residents with basic health training, traditional birth attendants, traditional healers	Recognition of signs and symptoms of abortion and complications Timely referral to the formal health care system
Primary	Health workers, nurses, trained midwives, general practitioners	All the above activities plus: — simple physical and pelvic examination — diagnosis of the stages of abortion — resuscitation and preparation for treatment or transfer — haematocrit/haemoglobin testing — referral, if needed *If trained staff and appropriate equipment are available, the following additional activities can be performed at this level:* — initiation of essential treatments including antibiotic therapy, intravenous fluid replacement, and oxytocics — uterine evacuation during the first trimester — basic pain control (paracervical block, simple analgesia and sedation)
First referral	Nurses, trained midwives, general practitioners, specialists with training in obstetrics and gynaecology	All of the above activities plus: — emergency uterine evacuation in the second trimester — treatment of most complications of abortion — blood cross-matching and transfusion — local and general anaesthesia — laparotomy and indicated surgery (including for ectopic pregnancy if skilled staff are available) — diagnosis and referral for severe complications such as septicaemia, peritonitis or renal failure
Secondary and tertiary	Nurses, trained midwives, general practitioners; obstetrics and gynaecology specialists	All of the above activities plus: — uterine evacuation as indicated — treatment of severe complications (including bowel injury, tetanus, renal failure, gas gangrene, severe sepsis) — treatment of coagulopathy

The aspects of emergency abortion care that should be available in the community, if there are trained health care workers at this level, include:

- recognition of the signs and symptoms of spontaneous abortion and abortion complications;
- timely referral to the formal health care system, as required.

Two additional preventive activities that may be performed at this level if workers have been trained are:

- provision of health education regarding unsafe abortion;
- provision of family planning information, education and services.

Primary level

Primary health care facilities, including first aid stations, nursing posts, dispensaries, health posts and centres, comprise the most basic level of the formal health care system. Basic health services, including health education, simple laboratory tests and treatment, are usually provided at this level. Inpatient care is not generally available. In addition, staff in these facilities may supervise community health activities such as those described above.

Primary health care facilities are seldom staffed by a full complement of health care professionals. At this level, there are often only limited staff and no persons trained to perform uterine evacuation. Training health care workers to provide emergency abortion care is a practical solution to staff shortages, particularly in developing countries where there may be few physicians and limited numbers of other medical staff. In a few countries, notably Bangladesh, Nigeria and Zaire, and in some states of the United States of America, non-physicians have been successfully trained to perform simple uterine evacuation for treatment of early, uncomplicated, incomplete abortion or for elective abortion (Begum et al., 1984, 1985; Freedman et al., 1986; Ladipo et al., 1978; Starrs, 1987).

Primary level facilities should generally have staff trained to provide the elements of emergency abortion care noted for the community level plus the following basic services:

- simple physical and pelvic examinations (especially vital signs and determination of uterine size);
- diagnosis of the stages of abortion;

- emergency resuscitation and preparation for treatment or transfer (including management of the airway and respiration, control of bleeding, control of pain);
- laboratory tests: haematocrit (erythrocyte volume fraction) and haemoglobin;
- referral (including arrangements for transportation) to first referral or higher level facilities for treatment of complications beyond the capability of this level.

When trained staff and equipment are available, a broader range of emergency abortion care services can be provided at the primary level thus making care more accessible to women. This extended range includes:

- initiation of essential treatment, including antibiotic therapy, intravenous fluid replacement, and oxytocics, as needed;
- uterine evacuation during the first trimester;
- basic pain control (paracervical block, simple analgesia) and sedation.

First referral level

When a woman's health care needs are beyond the capability of the primary health care facility, she should be transferred to a first referral facility. The first referral level is capable of providing some specialized services because more skilled personnel, equipment, medications, and emergency back-up services are available. First referral facilities are district or cottage hospitals with 20 or more beds providing inpatient services. Staff should be available at this level to provide services 24 hours a day. In some countries, specialized maternal and child health or maternity centres fulfil the criteria for first referral facilities.

Facilities at this level should have the trained staff and equipment necessary to carry out life-saving surgical and medical procedures for all except the most complicated cases. Staff at the first referral level usually include at least one physician. Physicians who can be trained in life-saving obstetric and gynaecological procedures may be available in some facilities. However, as noted on page 23, trained non-physicians may perform simple surgical procedures such as uterine evacuation, leaving doctors free to attend to more complicated procedures. Other reproductive health services provided at this level typically include caesarean section, surgical contraception, and elective abortion as allowed by local regulations (WHO, 1991).

First referral facilities should be equipped for and have trained staff who can provide all emergency abortion care activities noted for the community and primary levels, together with:

- emergency uterine evacuation as indicated during the second trimester;
- treatment of most abortion complications;
- blood cross-matching and transfusion;
- local and general anaesthesia;
- laparotomy and indicated surgery (including removal of ectopic pregnancy, if skilled staff are available);
- pregnancy testing;
- diagnosis of and referral (including arrangements for transportation) for major complications such as septicaemia, peritonitis, or renal failure, and any other cases that cannot be managed at the facility.

Secondary and tertiary levels

Secondary level facilities are full-service regional hospitals providing inpatient and outpatient services. University teaching hospitals and specialized national hospitals comprise the tertiary level. These facilities must be equipped and staffed to handle referrals on a 24-hours-a-day basis for all complicated emergency abortion cases. All services noted above for the community, primary, and first referral levels should be available at these levels, as well as:

- uterine evacuation as indicated;
- treatment of severe complications (including bowel injury, tetanus, renal failure, gas gangrene, severe sepsis);
- treatment of coagulopathy.

References

BEGUM SF ET AL. (1984) *A study on menstrual regulation providers in Bangladesh.* Dhaka, Bangladesh Association for Prevention of Septic Abortion.

BEGUM SF ET AL. (1985) *Evaluation of MR services and training programs.* Dhaka, Bangladesh Association for Prevention of Septic Abortion.

FLAHAULT D ET AL. (1988) *The supervision of health personnel at district level.* Geneva, World Health Organization.

FREEDMAN MA ET AL. (1986) Comparison of complication rates in first trimester abortions performed by physician assistants and physicians. *American journal of public health,* **76**(5): 550–554.

LADIPO OA ET AL. (1978) Menstrual regulation in Ibadan, Nigeria. *International journal of gynecology and obstetrics*, **15**(5): 428–432.

STARRS A (1987) *Preventing the tragedy of maternal deaths: a report on the International Safe Motherhood Conference*. Washington, DC, World Bank.

WHO (1985) *Prevention of maternal mortality. Report on a WHO Interregional Meeting*. Geneva, World Health Organization (unpublished document FHE/86.1; available on request from Division of Family Health, World Health Organization, 1211 Geneva 27, Switzerland).

WHO (1991) *Essential elements of obstetric care at first referral level*. Geneva, World Health Organization.

Chapter 3

LEGAL AND SOCIETAL FACTORS AFFECTING ABORTION CARE

> Abortion is more than a medical issue, or an ethical issue, or a legal issue. It is, above all, a human issue, involving women and men as individuals, as couples, and as members of societies (Tietze, 1978).

This chapter looks at existing laws and regulations on abortion and the ways in which legal and societal factors affect abortion behaviour and abortion care. The need for abortion care affects women from all social, economic, religious and cultural environments. Regardless of the constraints produced by the environment in which they live, it is clear that many women will seek induced abortion. The motivation to terminate pregnancy may compel a woman to deviate from long-held beliefs. This motivation can be so strong that women who are otherwise law-abiding and concerned about their health are willing to break the law and risk illness, death, and social and legal consequences to avert unwanted births (David et al., 1978).

Legal and societal factors also affect the interaction between women and health care workers, as well as the accessibility and quality of the care provided. Managers at all levels must have a clear understanding of the attitudes, beliefs and laws regarding abortion in the areas where they work in order to prevent these factors from hindering the provision of care. Emergency abortion care, in particular, should not be subject to regulations that are in any way different from those governing other medical and surgical procedures in the country.

Laws and regulations

Like all health care, abortion care is subject to regulations in the health code of any country. Professional training and licensing of health care providers, standards of medical practice, facilities, staffing, advertising, funding and fees for services are some of the aspects of health care that are commonly regulated.

Emergency abortion care

The provision of emergency abortion care is a requirement of the ethical practice of medicine in every country, as this care is often essential to save a woman's life and preserve health (Kleinman, 1988). Legal regulations, national medical norms and standards of practice usually determine how and where emergency abortion care may be delivered and who is qualified to provide it.

Elective abortion

The common practice of induced abortion is evident in all parts of the world throughout history, even in areas with legal prohibitions on abortion. In many countries, abortion is legal to preserve health.[1] Restrictions on the circumstances under which it may be provided vary widely. Henshaw & Morrow (1990) made the following estimates regarding laws on induced abortion (Fig. 2):

- 40% of the world's population live in countries where induced abortion is permitted on the request of the woman. Many countries have gestational limits, beyond which health or other indications are required.

- 23% of the world's population live in countries where sociomedical factors may be considered indications for induced abortion or where adverse social conditions alone can justify termination of pregnancy.

Fig. 2. Laws regarding abortion: percentage of the world's population affected, by category

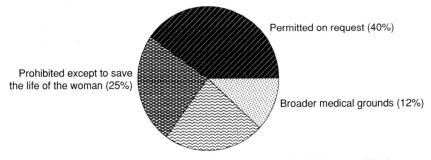

Permitted on request (40%)

Prohibited except to save the life of the woman (25%)

Broader medical grounds (12%)

Social or sociomedical indications (23%)

WHO 93538

Source: Henshaw & Morrow, 1990.

---

[1] As defined in the WHO Constitution, health is a state of complete physical, mental and social well-being and not merely the absence of disease or infirmity.

- 12% of the world's population live in countries where broad medical grounds, such as a threat to the woman's health or fetal indications justify termination of pregnancy.

- 25% of the world's population live in countries where induced abortion is prohibited except to save the life of the pregnant woman or without explicit exception.

The laws concerning abortion have changed over time, and modernization has generally been associated with liberalization of laws governing the provision of elective abortion. It is interesting to note that remnants of colonial law limiting the availability of induced abortion still exist in some countries such as Burkina Faso, Indonesia, Kenya, Mali, Nigeria, and many Latin American countries long after the laws have been liberalized in the former colonizing countries.

The revision or liberalization of abortion laws does not always lead immediately to improvements in abortion practice and safety and may not ensure access to services for women of all socioeconomic or cultural groups, or for women living in remote areas. For example, in some countries that liberalized their abortion laws some years ago, factors such as inadequate availability of services, lack of trained staff, and lack of information have limited the practice and availability of elective abortion. Unsafe abortions are still performed in these countries; thus, the need for emergency abortion care continues.

Legal restrictions on elective abortion can be changed and managers should be aware of the impact of any such changes on the services to be delivered. From the late 1960s to the late 1980s, changes in the law occurred in at least 69 jurisdictions, 65 being liberalizations and four limiting the grounds for abortion (Cook, 1989). Recent changes to abortion laws have defined new indications for the procedure, including adolescence, advanced maternal age, family circumstances and maternal infection with the human immunodeficiency virus (HIV).

Sociocultural and religious perspectives

The social and cultural environment in which a woman lives, the dominant religion, and her own personal beliefs all contribute to the decisions she makes regarding unintended pregnancy and the services she receives which, in turn, affect the mortality and morbidity associated with abortion. In addition, the socio-cultural perspectives and religious beliefs of health care workers affect their attitudes towards women who need abortion care and the services they provide. Some of the sociocultural elements that can affect abortion mortality and morbidity include:

- *Women's ability and willingness to seek care* promptly when they experience complications of abortion. Women may need their husbands' or guardians' permission to seek and use health services. For many women, an unintended pregnancy or use of abortion services can lead to social ostracism or rejection by family members. To avoid such rejection, women will often delay seeking care, even to the point of death. Health care workers must not contribute to this judgement of the woman. Rather, they must provide care which is accessible and supportive encouraging the woman to seek, rather than hide from, medical help.

- *Women's decision to seek to terminate a pregnancy and the sources and methods that they prefer.* Cultural factors may lead women to seek abortions that are dangerous. The reasons for these choices are many including trust in traditional providers, desire for secrecy, belief that non-medically induced abortions are not actual abortions, and referrals from family and friends.

- *Importance of fertility.* In many societies, a woman's fertility is central to her acceptance by the community. She may be unwilling to use modern contraception because she perceives it as harmful to her fertility. This behaviour increases her chances of unwanted pregnancy, and thus the risk of unsafe abortion.

- *Provider attitudes towards women's abortion care needs.* Studies have documented that women are unwilling to seek care from facilities that make them feel uncomfortable or where they have been treated badly (Bamisaiye, 1984; Feierman, 1981; Lasker, 1981; Thaddeus & Maine, 1990). It is particularly important that clinic and hospital staff are aware of and sympathetic to cultural factors when women from diverse cultural groups are cared for at the same facility.

Religion is an important factor in how women feel about their abortion experiences and how women who have abortions are treated by their communities. The importance of religious leaders in influencing people's attitudes about abortion and in combating community misinformation about fertility, abortion and family planning cannot be overestimated. For more details about informational needs, see Chapter 14.

Religious beliefs are also a factor in how staff providing emergency abortion care respond to patients and how those providing elective abortion view the services they provide. When a health care worker's personal religious beliefs interfere with the provision of legally sanctioned elective abortion, he or she should not be required to provide this service; however, he or she must be willing to make a prompt referral to another provider for this service.

Religious beliefs must never prevent the provision of life-saving emergency abortion care.

References

BAMISAIYE A (1984) Selected factors influencing the coverage of an MCH clinic in Lagos, Nigeria. *Journal of tropical pediatrics*, **30**(5): 256–261.

COOK RJ (1989) Abortion laws and policies: challenges and opportunities. In: Rosenfield A et al., eds. Women's health in the Third World: the impact of unwanted pregnancy. *International journal of gynecology and obstetrics*, Supplement 3: 61–87.

DAVID H ET AL., eds. (1978) *Abortion in psychosocial perspective: trends in transnational research*. New York, Springer.

FEIERMAN EK (1981) Alternative medical services in rural Tanzania: a physician's view. *Social science and medicine*, **15B**(3): 399–404.

HENSHAW SK, MORROW E (1990) *Induced abortion: a world review, 1990 supplement*. New York, Alan Guttmacher Institute.

KLEINMAN R, ed. (1988) *Family planning handbook for doctors*, 6th ed. London, International Planned Parenthood Federation.

LASKER JN (1981) Choosing among therapies: illness behavior in the Ivory Coast. *Social science and medicine*, **15A**(2): 157–168.

THADDEUS S, MAINE D (1990) *Too far to walk: maternal mortality in context*. New York, Columbia University Center for Population and Family Health.

TIETZE C (1978) Foreword. In: David H et al., eds. *Abortion in psychosocial perspective: trends in transnational research*. New York, Springer.

PLANNING FOR ABORTION CARE

Systematic planning accounts for the difference between health services that work and those that do not (Rogo, 1990).

The remaining chapters of these guidelines review the major programme elements or tasks required in the planning and provision of abortion care and the managerial requirements of each task. The following list summarizes the tasks and indicates the chapters in which additional information about each can be found:

- planning for abortion care (Chapter 4);
- clinical aspects of emergency abortion care (Chapters 5–7);
- patient counselling and informational needs (Chapter 8);
- management of facilities and equipment (Chapter 9);
- skill requirements, training and supervision of personnel (Chapter 10);
- decentralization and coordination of care, referral and transportation (Chapter 11);
- monitoring, evaluation and information systems (Chapter 12);
- cost and financing issues in abortion care (Chapter 13);
- preventive measures to reduce unsafe abortion (Chapter 14).

Strategic planning

Planning is an essential component of the delivery of all types of health services, including abortion care. Following a logical planning sequence is crucial to ensure successful services and to maintain their safety, effectiveness and efficiency. Inadequate planning often results in wasted time and money and in poorly designed services which do not meet the needs of the population. Conversely, careful planning contributes to provision of services of the highest quality possible as well as increased efficiency in the use of resources. These are important factors for the ultimate achievement of the goal of reduced maternal mortality and morbidity.

Planning is comprised of the following steps:

(*a*) identifying a problem and defining its scope;

(*b*) setting programme objectives;

(*c*) determining the interventions (steps, strategies or activities) needed to achieve the objectives;

(*d*) monitoring and evaluating programme implementation and impact.

Steps (*a*)–(*c*) are described below. Step (*d*) is discussed in Chapter 12.

Problem identification and definition

The mere perception of problems in delivery of abortion care is sufficient reason to look for ways to improve services. Nevertheless, it is important to identify the problems and assess their scope by delineating the gap between what is needed and what is currently available. This step is sometimes called a needs assessment, situational analysis, or environmental analysis.

Needs assessment consists of the collection of relevant information or data, and analysis of the data to obtain an accurate understanding of the situation. While surveys and formal studies are useful when resources are available, collection of information does not have to be done through a lengthy, costly research effort. Useful information can be gained simply by reviewing existing records and talking with staff and members of the community. Information about existing health services, potential caseload, the scope of services needed, the general health goals of the locality, and relevant laws of the jurisdiction can be collected from formal and informal sources.

Tables 6 and 7 indicate the information that can be collected to assist in planning abortion care, the sources of this information, and its possible uses. Collecting the information as noted in these tables from the sources listed is the ideal. However, the delivery of necessary emergency abortion care should not be postponed simply because some of this information is unavailable.

Table 6. Health care system information, sources and uses

Types of information	Potential sources								Suggested uses
	Patient records	Quality assurance reports	Inventory records	Financial records	Health training institutions	Personnel records	Interviews	Standard operating procedures	
Description of the health care system									To determine general potential for abortion care services by level and facility
Staff (including training)					X	X	X	X	To determine staff training needs
Equipment			X				X		To determine equipment and supply needs
Supplies			X				X		
Abortion care services provided	X						X	X	
Current and potential abortion caseload	X						X		To plan and budget for abortion care services
									To establish objectives
Complications/mortality rates	X	X					X		To determine training needs
									To review existing legislation
Cost of emergency abortion care	X			X					To assist in budget development
									To review existing legislation
Quality of care (adequacy of clinical services, space availability, patient flow, waiting time, patients' perceptions, etc.)	X	X	X				X	X	To improve the delivery of high-quality abortion care

Table 7. National and community information, sources and uses

Types of information	Potential sources						Suggested uses
	Census	Special surveys	Hospital records	Government records	Abortion registries	Interviews	
Population/demographic data							
No. of women of reproductive age	X	X					To determine target groups and potential caseload
Birth rates	X	X					To determine trends in birth and maternal mortality rates as indicators of the demand for abortion
Maternal mortality rates (by cause)	X	X	X	X	X		
Sociocultural and religious beliefs		X				X	To design educational activities and services
Legal and political status of abortion				X			To design services and record-keeping and determine reporting requirements
Reproductive patterns/activities		X		X	X	X	To determine knowledge, attitudes and practices of abortion and family planning To determine trends To determine unmet demand
Economic indicators							
Women's participation in the labour force	X	X				X	To determine economic impact of abortion mortality and morbidity
Cost of abortion and family planning		X	X			X	To determine willingness to pay for services and the amount to charge, if applicable

Table 7 (continued)

Types of information	Census	Special surveys	Hospital records	Government records	Abortion registries	Interviews	Suggested uses
				Potential sources			
Community resources							
Current abortion and family planning providers		X			X	X	To determine availability and safety of current services
Availability of resources for abortion care		X	X	X		X	To develop a budget, and referral and educational systems for abortion care
Potential collaborators (referral and educational resources)		X		X		X	

Setting objectives

Managers need to set specific programme objectives aimed at reducing abortion mortality and morbidity, and based on an understanding of the needs for emergency abortion care and the status of existing services. Programme objectives should indicate the specific changes that managers expect the programme to achieve within a given time period. Some examples of programme objectives for abortion care are as follows:

- to train all professional midwives at the primary level to perform first-trimester emergency uterine evacuation, within four years;
- to treat 75% of women with abortion complications at the first referral level, rather than referring them to higher levels, within one year;
- to supply written information about the dangers of unsafe abortion and prevention of unwanted pregnancy to at least 80% of high school students within two years.

Part of the process of setting objectives is the development of "benchmarks" or indicators of progress towards their achievement, which will enable managers to monitor the programme. Benchmarks should be as specific as possible and a target completion date should be established. For example, if the objective is to train professional midwives at the primary care level to perform first-trimester emergency uterine evacuation within four years, some important benchmarks would be:

- to establish a training curriculum during the first three months;
- to hold regular training sessions for new midwives coming to primary health care centres each year;
- to conduct a follow-up assessment of midwives' skills at primary health care facilities after training is completed;
- to evaluate the training programme after four years.

Interventions

Interventions are the activities implemented to meet the programme objectives. Interventions to improve abortion care can take place at all levels, from the national health care system to individual facilities. Interventions may include the following.

At the national level

- Revising the curricula used in the training of health professionals to include emergency abortion care.
- Decentralizing emergency abortion care to primary health care centres.
- Adding elective abortion care as an outpatient procedure at the lowest appropriate level of care in response to changes in legislation or policy.
- Changing the list of equipment and supplies recommended for purchase in support of introduction of an improved procedure.

At the subnational (e.g. provincial, state, zone) level

- Training traditional practitioners to provide health education about family planning and the dangers of unsafe abortion.
- Holding a conference for health planners and managers to present data about the impact of complications of unsafe abortion on use of health care resources.
- Conducting seminars to improve the efficiency of referral and transport between levels of care.

At the hospital or clinic level

- Establishing a treatment room for emergency abortion care in the outpatient clinic or casualty ward.
- Changing from dilatation and curettage (D&C) to vacuum aspiration for abortion care.
- Instituting standards and monitoring infection control practices, including disposal of waste and cleaning of equipment for all staff.
- Holding in-service training sessions for staff about clinical and psychosocial issues in abortion care.
- Shifting delivery of elective abortion services to an outpatient service.
- Decreasing use of general anaesthesia for uterine evacuation.

At the community level

- Training village health workers to recognize abortion complications, and to refer patients for emergency abortion care.

● Teaching village health workers about the need to avoid unsafe abortion practices.

Reference

Rogo K (1990) *Medical implications and adolescent sexuality.* Paper presented at the First Inter-African Conference on Adolescent Health, Nairobi.

Chapter 5

INITIAL ASSESSMENT IN EMERGENCY ABORTION CARE

In addition to the general health of the individual woman, four major factors determine the mortality and morbidity from both legal and illegal abortion—the skill of the provider, the duration of the pregnancy, and the accessibility and quality of medical facilities to treat complications of abortion (Liskin, 1980).

Because of the frequency with which complications of both spontaneous and induced abortion occur, facilities at every level of the health care system must be able to provide basic elements of emergency abortion care. The specific services provided at a particular facility or by any given health care worker range from health education, resuscitation, and referral to surgical intervention for severe complications.

This chapter provides information about assessment of the condition of women seeking care for incomplete abortion and the treatment of severe complications that require immediate attention. Chapter 6 provides information on uterine evacuation techniques for the removal of retained products of conception, a procedure that is required for the vast majority of women seeking emergency abortion care, and that is also the central element of elective abortion services. It is essential for managers at all levels to be familiar with this information in order to determine facility requirements, equipment and supply needs, staffing patterns, and training needs. All of these topics are covered in more detail in later chapters.

Initial assessment

Women seeking advice or treatment for unexpected bleeding, fever or lower abdominal pain may or may not know whether they are pregnant. In either case, they could be experiencing a spontaneous abortion or complications of abortion. Therefore, whenever a health care worker at any level of the health care system is consulted by a woman of reproductive age with these symptoms, the possibility of pregnancy should be considered regardless of the woman's menstrual or contraceptive history.

An accurate initial assessment is essential to ensure appropriate treatment or prompt referral.

The critical signs and symptoms of incomplete abortion and the complications that require immediate attention include:

- vaginal bleeding,
- abdominal pain,
- infection,
- shock.

Personnel at all levels of the health care system must be able to take a brief medical history and assess the woman's immediate physical condition. It may be difficult for health care workers with little training and limited resources to diagnose incomplete abortion and its complications with certainty. A life-threatening condition such as extrauterine or ectopic pregnancy may produce a positive pregnancy test and symptoms similar to those of incomplete abortion, thus compounding the difficulty of making a definite diagnosis. It is essential, therefore, for health care personnel to be prepared to make referrals and arrange transport to a facility where a definitive diagnosis can be made and appropriate care can be delivered quickly.

If trained, the personnel at the first point of contact should perform a physical examination including measurement of temperature, pulse and blood pressure (vital signs), as well as a pelvic examination (speculum and bimanual). If the physical examination does not reveal clear evidence of pregnancy, laboratory confirmation of pregnancy is desirable. If such confirmation is not possible, treatment must proceed on the basis of the history and clinical findings alone. An evaluation of the duration and amount of bleeding and an estimate of gestational age[1] and uterine size by palpation are required. If foul or purulent vaginal discharge is present, an appropriate specimen may be obtained for laboratory diagnosis where feasible, but should not delay the initiation of treatment.

Spontaneous abortion is a frequent occurrence and may happen before pregnancy is recognized or diagnosed (Wilcox et al., 1988). The diagnostic categories and management of spontaneous abortion are presented in Table 8. Uncomplicated

---

[1] Throughout this text, all references to gestation or the length of pregnancy are based on the number of completed weeks since the first day of the last menstrual period.

Table 8. Clinical management of uncomplicated spontaneous abortion

Diagnosis	Findings	Treatment[a]
Threatened abortion	Slight or moderate bleeding Cramps Cervix not dilated Positive pregnancy test	Observation Reduced activity
Inevitable abortion	Bleeding Cervix dilated	Observation Uterine evacuation Uterotonic drugs
Incomplete abortion	Bleeding Partial expulsion of products of conception Cervix dilated	Uterine evacuation without delay Uterotonic drugs
Complete abortion	Complete expulsion of products of conception	Observation Uterotonic drugs
Missed abortion	Fetal demise with delayed expulsion May be complicated by afibrinogenaemia, dissemi- nated intravascular coagula- tion, severe bleeding Uterus small for dates Regression of pregnancy	Uterine evacuation as soon as possible May require treatment for coagulopathy

[a] All treatment including use of uterotonics by non-physician personnel should be guided by local treatment protocols.

spontaneous abortion can be treated on an outpatient basis at the primary level if trained staff and appropriate equipment are available. Women treated for uncomplicated spontaneous abortion can usually be discharged after a short period of observation. When a woman seeks care at a facility that is not equipped or staffed to provide the care needed, stabilization and prompt referral for care are essential.

When referral to a higher level of care is required, clinic staff should be able to resuscitate patients (i.e., to restore or maintain vital signs) so that they can be transported without delay to the nearest referral facility for definitive treatment (see Chapter 11). The following basic elements of emergency resuscitation should be available without delay wherever women initially seek care, especially in preparation for referral and transport or when definitive management is delayed:

● management of the airway and respiration;
● control of bleeding;

- intravenous fluid replacement;
- control of pain.

Complications of abortion requiring emergency care

The major life-threatening complications resulting from unsafe abortion are haemorrhage, infection, and injury to the genital tract and internal organs. Retained products of conception often contribute to these complications; this topic is covered in Chapter 6. Toxic reactions to chemicals and drugs used to induce abortion may add to the complications among women who ultimately seek care from the formal health system. Health care services at all levels must be available 24 hours a day to provide emergency care for these complications in line with their capabilities.

Two important observations have emerged in studies of all types of abortion complications:

- the occurrence of morbidity and mortality is directly proportional to gestational age;
- complications are more frequent and more severe in environments where self-induced or otherwise unsafe abortions are common and where family planning services to prevent unwanted pregnancy and safe clinical facilities for abortion care are lacking.

Accordingly, at the community level, education of health care workers and the general public to encourage early and safe management of spontaneous and induced abortion and decreased use of unsafe practices is a first line of prevention of complications.

Management of haemorrhage

Prolonged or excessive bleeding is the most common complication seen in abortion care services. Retained products of conception are the main cause of bleeding in most abortion cases, but trauma or damage from chemical agents, or complications of blood coagulation in cases of missed abortion, can also be the cause. If retained products of conception are the reason for the haemorrhage, the uterus should be evacuated. However, if cervical trauma or damage is the cause, the lesion should be sutured. Non-surgical procedures to stop bleeding include uterine massage and administration of uterotonic drugs.

Timely treatment of excessive blood loss is critical in abortion care, as delays in controlling haemorrhage and replacing fluid or blood volume can be fatal. Blood loss can be assessed by measuring blood pressure, pulse rate, and urine flow. After initial assessment and intravenous fluid replacement, referral as soon as possible to a facility with equipment and supplies for blood transfusion may be indicated. Arrangements for referral, including transportation, should be pre-established to minimize delay. For more information on referral networks, see Chapter 11.

Selective use of transfusions of blood or blood products is important to reduce the risk of transmitting infectious agents such as hepatitis or human immunodeficiency virus. Acute blood loss should usually be managed through the use of normal saline and plasma expanders rather than packed red blood cells or whole blood. In most cases, replacement of blood volume rather than of red blood cells is needed, and plasma expanders are safer, less expensive and can be transfused faster. Only women who have both a low haemoglobin level and symptoms of acute blood loss or severe anaemia should receive transfusions (Hollán et al., 1990). For information on materials required for blood transfusion, see Annex 2G.

Where blood transfusion is required appropriate precautions should be taken. The Global Blood Safety Initiative, a collaborative effort of WHO and several other international agencies, has produced guidelines for the appropriate use of blood. These guidelines provide specific information regarding the management of haemorrhage and shock and the arrangements required for administration of blood and blood components. The guidelines should be studied by managers at all levels and made available to the staff at all facilities involved in blood replacement (WHO, 1989). Blood that has not been obtained from appropriately selected donors, or that has not been screened for infectious agents, should not be transfused other than in the most exceptional life-threatening situations (WHO, 1989).

Management of infection

Infection in abortion patients should be suspected if the woman has any of the following symptoms:

- fever and chills,
- foul-smelling vaginal or cervical discharge,
- pain in the abdomen or pelvis,

- prolonged bleeding or spotting,
- tenderness of the uterus and adnexa during pelvic examination or pain with cervical motion.

These patients require antibiotic therapy along with evacuation of the uterine contents as soon as possible (see Chapter 6). Treatment is best accomplished on an inpatient basis, but can sometimes be managed on an outpatient basis, depending on the severity of the infection, the patient's ability to adhere to the treatment regimen, and her willingness and ability to use follow-up care. If severe infection has spread beyond the uterus or if septicaemia is diagnosed, hospitalization is required, and specific laboratory diagnosis, intravenous fluids, parenteral antibiotic therapy, intensive care, and sometimes additional surgery may be required. In particular, the occurrence of septic shock, a life-threatening condition involving circulatory collapse caused by a bacterial toxin, requires intensive medical management at a higher level facility.

Infection rarely follows a safe elective abortion but when it occurs is most often associated with retained products of conception in the uterus. In this instance, the signs of infection may not appear until several days after the procedure. Accordingly, all patients must be informed of the importance of recognizing and reporting such symptoms as fever, pain, and foul-smelling vaginal discharge. Treatment depends on the severity of infection. In mild cases, orally administered broad-spectrum antibiotics and re-evacuation of the uterus generally suffice.

The value of prophylactic antibiotics in abortion care has been demonstrated in a number of studies. Their routine use must be determined by local availability and practice. In any case, their use is strongly recommended in individuals considered to be at high risk of infection: those with a history of pelvic inflammatory disease, with multiple sexual partners, or who have undergone an unsafe induced abortion. Use of tetanus toxoid and tetanus antitoxin should also be based on local needs and policy.

Management of injury to the genital tract and internal organs

Injury to the genital tract and internal organs is a life-threatening complication as well as a cause of serious long-term morbidity among abortion patients. Whenever an injury is diagnosed, accurate recording of the woman's condition is important for possible future interventions and postoperative observation. Most often these injuries occur if the attempted abortion has been performed by an unqualified person or has been self-induced. Occasionally, trauma may occur in procedures performed in a medical setting by a trained health care worker. Almost any internal organ can be damaged. The most common injuries are uterine perforation and cervical lacerations. Damage to the ovaries, fallopian tubes, bladder, bowel, and rectum can also occur.

The cervix may be damaged through the use of inappropriate instruments or through over-forceful dilatation. If uterine perforation is suspected, appropriate steps may include observation, laparoscopy or laparotomy. Any internal injury, if not readily diagnosed and treated, can lead to serious complications including bleeding, infection and, ultimately, death. Therefore, whenever a woman is treated for complications following an unsafe abortion, the possibility of a life-threatening genital tract injury should be considered. When indicated, early referral to an appropriate level of care for comprehensive management is critical. Even with treatment, the woman's health status and future fertility may be greatly jeopardized in these cases.

Management of toxic and chemical reactions

Systemic and localized reactions can result from drugs and other chemicals used to induce abortion. Symptoms vary greatly depending on the particular substance used and method of application. These substances are often used in combination with other, usually traumatic, abortion techniques. Thus, women diagnosed with haemorrhage, infection or trauma should be assessed for toxic chemical and drug reactions as well. Possible effects include damage to the liver and kidneys, gastrointestinal upset, central nervous system effects such as headache, confusion, and delirium, and chemical burns. If signs of a chemical burn are present, special care should be taken to avoid infection, fluid loss and dehydration. The long-term effects of chemical burns include scarring and stenosis.

Management of failed evacuation

It is essential, in both emergency and induced abortion care, to ensure that there are no products of conception left in the uterus. Failed evacuation may occur with any uterine evacuation procedure, whether for treatment of abortion complications or for induction of abortion. In emergency abortion care, it is difficult to know what quantity of products to expect. It is therefore always extremely important to inspect the evacuated tissue. With induced abortion, the pregnancy may not be interrupted, especially in cases of very early gestation (5–7 weeks) or cases of uterine anomalies or distortions. Absence of fetal parts or placental elements in tissue obtained in uterine evacuation (see Chapter 7) could indicate failed evacuation and an ongoing pregnancy or ectopic pregnancy, both of which require further investigation and prompt treatment. Re-evacuation of the uterus may be necessary in the case of failed evacuation. Such occurrences underscore the importance of careful explanation of discharge instructions regarding complications and resumption of menses (see page 58).

Long-term sequelae of unsafe abortion

Unsafe abortion is a major cause of maternal morbidity. On the other hand, safe induced abortion has not generally been associated with harmful long-term sequelae. Reliance on unskilled abortionists operating in unhygienic conditions or efforts to induce abortion themselves leave many women with grave physical impairment, pain, pelvic inflammatory disease (PID), secondary infertility, and increased risk of ectopic pregnancy. Women with a history of PID are at high risk of post-abortion pelvic infection and its consequences, impaired fertility and pelvic pain (Heisterberg, 1988). The morbidity directly associated with unsafely induced abortion is compounded by the inadequate emergency care available to many women and the delays in receiving care.

References

HEISTERBERG L (1988) Pelvic inflammatory disease following induced first-trimester abortion. *Danish medical bulletin*, **35**(1): 64–75.

HOLLÁN SR ET AL., eds (1990) *Management of blood transfusion services.* Geneva, World Health Organization.

LISKIN LS (1980) Complications of abortion in developing countries. *Population reports*, Series F, No. 7.

WILCOX AJ ET AL. (1988) Incidence of early loss of pregnancy. *New England journal of medicine*, **319**(4): 189–242.

WHO (1989) *Global Blood Safety Initiative: Guidelines for the appropriate use of blood.* Geneva, World Health Organization (unpublished document WHO/LAB/89.10; available from Health Laboratory Technology and Blood Safety, World Health Organization, 1211 Geneva 27, Switzerland).

WHO (1990) *Core protocol of the operational research study on adequate supply of blood at the community or first referral level.* Geneva, World Health Organization (unpublished document, available from Maternal and Child Health and Family Planning, World Health Organization, 1211 Geneva 27, Switzerland).

Chapter 6

METHODS OF UTERINE EVACUATION

Existing technologies have been improved and new ones developed for safe and effective methods of uterine evacuation; some drugs are emerging as potentially effective abortifacients. To assist women with abortion complications, and to reduce the incidence of complications, it is essential that clinicians have access to and acquire skills to use these safe, cost-effective technologies (Ladipo, 1989).

Uterine evacuation, or the complete removal of the products of conception, is essential for both emergency and elective abortion care. In emergency abortion care this procedure should be accomplished without delay to reduce complications, especially in cases of profuse or prolonged bleeding. Uterine evacuation can be made widely available, since elaborate facilities are not required. WHO includes uterine evacuation for incomplete abortion as one of the essential elements of obstetric care that should be available at the first referral level (WHO, 1991). In addition, in many countries uterine evacuation is available at the primary health care level, where trained health care workers sometimes perform the procedure.

Many techniques are available for uterine evacuation. Generally, the techniques used at any given level of the health care system are based on the clinical indications, the skill and experience of staff at the facility, and the availability of specific equipment and drugs. Limits on gestational age or uterine size that can be managed at a specific facility may vary according to local norms and preferences. However, the guiding principles for surgical evacuation of the uterus include strict asepsis and complete removal of products of conception with minimal trauma, regardless of the level of service at which care is given or the technique used.

First-trimester emergency methods

First-trimester abortions are defined as abortions taking place at any time up to 12 completed weeks of pregnancy. The techniques of uterine evacuation used for emergency abortion care in the first trimester are as follows:

- *Vacuum aspiration.*[1] This is a minor gynaecological procedure involving minimum trauma, and is generally preferred for first-trimester uterine evacuation (Hodgson, 1981). Cannulae used for vacuum aspiration are made of flexible plastic, rigid plastic, or metal. Gentle exploration with a curette to confirm complete removal of the uterine contents may be employed after vacuum evacuation, but is not generally necessary or recommended. Vacuum sources for aspiration are manual syringes, electric pumps, and foot-operated mechanical pumps.
  - *Manual vacuum aspiration* requires a hand-held vacuum syringe and flexible plastic cannulae of various diameters (Fig. 3). This technique is usually limited to use when the uterine size does not exceed that corresponding to 12 weeks' gestation.
  - *Electric or foot-operated mechanical pumps* can be used with either plastic or metal cannulae. Use of these pumps is sometimes extended to the early part of the second trimester.

- *Dilatation and curettage (D&C).* Curettage is still used in many areas; however, use of D&C is declining in favour of vacuum aspiration, which is safer and less traumatic if the equipment is available and well maintained.

Clinical research over the past 25 years has established vacuum aspiration as the safest technique for uterine evacuation for both incomplete and induced abortion in the first trimester. Over 70 studies involving more than 500 000 women document the safety and effectiveness of the technique (Greenslade et al, 1993).

The largest and most comprehensive study of vacuum aspiration, the Joint Program for the Study of Abortion (JPSA), analysed data from almost 250 000 induced abortion cases in the United States of America (Tietze & Lewit, 1972; Cates et al, 1977; Cates et al, 1979b; Buehler et al, 1975; Binkin, 1986; Tietze & Henshaw, 1986). The rates of major complications were lowest when vacuum aspiration was performed within 12 weeks of the last menstrual period. Abortions performed within 7–8 weeks

---

[1] Also called suction curettage, menstrual regulation (MR), endometrial aspiration, interception of pregnancy, and mini-suction.

Fig. 3.   Vacuum aspiration equipment

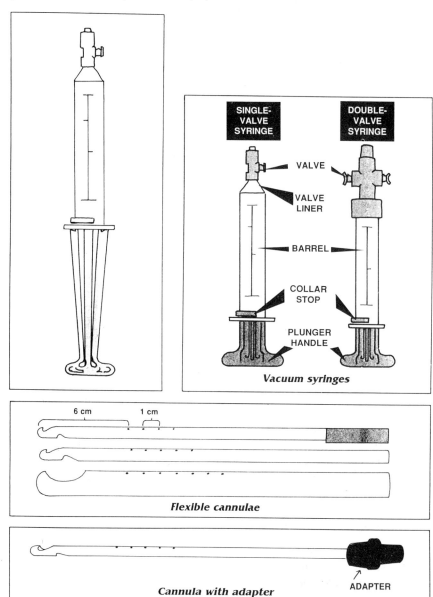

Vacuum syringes

Flexible cannulae

Cannula with adapter

ADAPTER

WHO 92590

had the lowest complication rates; the risk of major complications increased by 15–30% with each week of delay. Table 9 contains summary data from the JPSA, showing lower complication rates for vacuum aspiration than for sharp curettage for uterine evacuation.

Table 9. Comparison of complication rates of vacuum aspiration and sharp curettage

Procedure	Total no. of complications (per 100 abortions)	No. of major complications (per 100 abortions)
Vacuum aspiration	5.0	0.4
Sharp curettage	10.6	0.9

Adapted from Grimes et al., 1977a.

Early second-trimester emergency methods

Uterine evacuation up to 12–14 completed weeks of pregnancy can be performed safely in outpatient facilities if the facility has trained staff, suitable equipment and functioning referral links to nearby higher levels of care. Evacuation may be accomplished either by vacuum aspiration using an electric or foot-operated pump with large cannulae or by curettage (see page 49).

Late second-trimester emergency methods

Women diagnosed with incomplete abortion late in the second trimester of pregnancy (more than 14 completed weeks of pregnancy) should be treated at the first referral level. In most of these cases, the cervix is already dilated and the essential steps are to stop the bleeding and evacuate the uterus. This can be done by administering intravenous oxytocin and removing the uterine contents digitally or using instruments. The woman's condition, especially the occurrence of complications, may necessitate referral to a higher level of care.

First-trimester elective procedures

During the first trimester, the methods used for emergency uterine evacuation (vacuum aspiration or dilatation and curettage) can be used for elective abortion. In addition, the following techniques are worthy of note.

● *Menstrual regulation* (MR). This term refers to use of the manual vacuum aspiration technique using a hand-held syringe in very early pregnancy and sometimes refers to uterine evacuation when pregnancy has not been confirmed.

● *Anti-progestins.* Drugs such as mifepristone offer a promising new approach to early induced abortion. These orally administered synthetic drugs may provide a medical substitute for surgical evacuation, particularly when followed within 48 hours by administration of a prostaglandin. However, medical supervision is required owing to the possibility of prolonged or excessive bleeding, and the small but important risk of incomplete abortion or continuing pregnancy. Surgical completion of the evacuation may be needed in some cases.

Second-trimester elective procedures

Elective abortion beyond 14 weeks' gestation requires fully equipped surgical facilities and a higher level of operative skill owing to the greater potential for surgical trauma and excessive blood loss. The well-documented fact that complications of abortion increase in proportion to gestational age underscores the importance of creating an environment in which early termination of pregnancy is readily available in jurisdictions where legally allowed (Cates & Grimes, 1981). Uterine evacuation procedures late in the second trimester should be performed only where skilled providers and back-up facilities are available.

Methods used for such procedures vary but can include the following:

- *Dilatation and evacuation* (*D&E*). Surgical evacuation, using suction in combination with special forceps, has been shown to be safer than all other methods of abortion in the second trimester when performed by an experienced operator and when combined with the use of multiple laminaria tents or synthetic dilators (Cates et al., 1982; Grimes et al., 1977b; Peterson et al., 1983). A skilled operator and well equipped facility are essential (Cates et al., 1980).

- *Prostaglandins or prostaglandin derivatives.* These drugs may be used effectively either by intra-amniotic, extra-amniotic or vaginal administration. Use of prostaglandins may produce side-effects, some of which can be serious, requiring the patient to be admitted to a facility for medical supervision or observation (Cates et al., 1979a; Grimes et al., 1977c; Hern, 1990; Rogo & Nyamu, 1989). Other methods are considered safer.

- *Amnio-infusion of other products.* Substances such as hypertonic urea or saline are sometimes used to induce uterine contractions in the second trimester. These may produce side-effects, some of which can be serious. Amnio-infusion should generally be used with methods to soften the cervix such as multiple laminaria tents or prostaglandin suppositories.

- *Abdominal operative removal.* Hysterotomy and hysterectomy were once widely used for abortion in late pregnancy; however, these methods have been discredited and are now rarely used.

Cervical dilatation

Evacuation of the uterus requires that the cervix be sufficiently dilated to allow insertion of instruments. In some cases of incomplete abortion this degree of dilatation has already occurred when the treatment is begun and no further dilatation is required. In other cases the cervix must be further dilated, particularly when large instruments must enter the uterus. With induced abortion, some dilatation of the cervix is often required. Various methods are available including mechanical dilators (e.g., Pratt, Denniston, and Hegar dilators) and osmotic dilators (e.g., laminaria and synthetic substitutes). In procedures in late pregnancy, prostaglandin preparations are sometimes used to soften the cervix.

Whenever cervical dilatation is required it is important to minimize trauma to the cervix. A slow, gentle technique should be used with mechanical dilators. Paracervical block may be required to minimize the pain associated with mechanical dilatation.

References

Binkin NJ (1986) Trends in induced legal abortion morbidity and mortality. *Clinics in obstetrics and gynaecology*, **13**(1): 83–93.

Buehler JW et al. (1985) The risk of serious complications from induced abortion: do personal characteristics make a difference? *American journal of obstetrics and gynecology*, **153**(1): 14–20.

Cates W Jr, Grimes DA (1981) Morbidity and mortality in the United States. In: Hodgson JE, ed. *Abortion and sterilization: medical and social aspects.* London, Academic Press.

Cates W Jr et al. (1977) The effect of delay and method choice on the risk of abortion morbidity. *Family planning perspectives*, **9**(6): 266–273.

Cates W Jr et al. (1979a) Sudden collapse and death of women obtaining abortions induced with prostaglandin F2α. *American journal of obstetrics and gynecology,* **133**(4): 398–400.

Cates W Jr et al. (1979b) Short-term complications of uterine evacuation techniques for abortion at 12 weeks' gestation or earlier. In: Zatuchni GI, Sciarra JJ, Spiedel JJ, eds., *Pregnancy termination: procedures, safety and new developments.* Hagerstown, MD, Harper & Row.

CATES W Jr ET AL. (1980) Dilatation and evacuation for induced abortion in developing countries: advantages and disadvantages. *Studies in family planning,* **11**(4): 128–133.

CATES W Jr ET AL. (1982) Dilatation and evacuation procedures and second-trimester abortions: the role of physician skill and hospital setting. *Journal of the American Medical Association,* **248**(5): 559–563.

GREENSLADE FG ET AL. (1993) *Manual vacuum aspiration: a summary of clinical and programmatic experience worldwide.* Carrboro, NC, IPAS, 1993.

GRIMES DA ET AL. (1977a) The Joint Program for the Study of Abortion/CDC: a preliminary report. In: Hern W, Andrikopoulos B, eds. *Abortion in the seventies.* New York, National Abortion Federation.

GRIMES DA ET AL. (1977b) Mid-trimester abortion by dilatation and evacuation: a safe and practical alternative. *New England journal of medicine,* **296**(20): 1141–1145.

GRIMES DA ET AL. (1977c) Mid-trimester abortion by intraamniotic prostaglandin F2α: safer than saline? *Obstetrics and gynecology,* **49**(5): 612–616.

HERN WM (1990) *Abortion practice.* Philadelphia, Lippincott.

HODGSON JE, ed. (1981) *Abortion and sterilization: medical and social aspects.* London, Academic Press.

LADIPO OA (1989) Preventing and managing complications of induced abortion in Third World countries. In: Rosenfield A et al., eds. Women's health in the Third World: the impact of unwanted pregnancy. *International journal of gynecology and obstetrics,* Suppl. 3: 21–28.

PETERSON WF ET AL. (1983) Second-trimester abortion by dilatation and evacuation: an analysis of 11,747 cases. *Obstetrics and gynecology,* **62**(2): 185–190.

ROGO KO, NYAMU JM (1989) Legal termination of pregnancy at the Kenyatta National Hospital using prostaglandin F2α in mid-trimester. *East African medical journal,* **66**(5): 333–339.

TIETZE C, HENSHAW SK (1986) *Induced abortion: a world review, 1986.* New York, Alan Guttmacher Institute.

TIETZE C, LEWIT S (1972) Joint Program for the Study of Abortion (JPSA): early medical complications of legal abortion. *Studies in family planning,* **3**(6): 97–119.

WHO (1991) *Essential elements of obstetric care at first referral level.* Geneva, World Health Organization.

Chapter 7

ADDITIONAL CLINICAL ELEMENTS OF ABORTION CARE

A responsive reproductive health care strategy would attend to the reproductive health needs of all, by providing education for responsible and safe sex life, contraception for the sexually active to use as needed, and services for the management of pregnancy, delivery and all abortions (Sai & Nassim, 1989).

This chapter highlights elements of service delivery that are essential to the safety and effectiveness of care regardless of the method of uterine evacuation used. It is the responsibility of managers to see that these elements are included in service protocols and followed in practice by the staff.

Anaesthesia, sedation and analgesia

While general, regional and local anaesthesia have all been used in abortion care, local anaesthesia should suffice for the majority of uterine evacuation procedures. There are several advantages to using local anaesthesia compared with general anaesthesia. When a local anaesthetic is used, the patient remains alert and responsive and thus she can tell the provider if she experiences symptoms that could indicate a complication. The patient's alertness also allows the provider to continue supportive communication throughout the procedure which can minimize the need for further anaesthesia or sedation. In addition, recovery time is shorter when local anaesthesia is used (Nasser, 1989).

Anaesthesia, sedation and analgesia in emergency abortion care

The value of anaesthesia rather than analgesia in preventing pain and suffering during emergency abortion care must be weighed against its risks. Resuscitation of the patient must take precedence over preparation for and use of anaesthesia. Furthermore, patients with emergency complications of abortion may have conditions that place them at a higher risk of complications from anaesthesia, such as shock owing to blood loss, or sepsis (King, 1986).

The use of general or regional anaesthesia should be limited to institutions that have staff trained in their administration and, even in those institutions, should be used only when deemed necessary on an individual basis. It is important to evaluate the existence of conditions that contraindicate use of anaesthesia or affect the choice of anaesthetic and, to the extent possible, correct these conditions before administering anaesthesia. Certain anaesthetic gases, such as halothane or diethyl ether, can cause uterine relaxation and increased bleeding, and should be avoided if possible (Marx, 1978). Regional anaesthesia must be avoided in cases of haemorrhagic shock or coagulation problems (Dobson, 1988). Equipment for continuous intravenous infusion, tracheal intubation, oxygen administration and resuscitation is required if general or regional anaesthesia is to be used.

Paracervical block is useful in reducing the pain associated with cervical dilatation. A local anaesthetic is injected beneath the cervical mucosa at several positions around the cervix (Darney, 1987).

Sedation and non-narcotic analgesia can be employed, separately or in combination, to allay anxiety or to reduce the pain of uterine evacuation. In many instances, particularly in the first trimester and when the cervix is already dilated prior to the procedure, medication may not be needed. Decisions regarding the need for pain relief and the type to use should be individualized according to the woman's medical history, length of gestation, parity, perceived pain threshold, and level of anxiety, as well as the clinical resources of the facility.

Reassurance in advance of the procedure, supportive counselling, and the presence of a sympathetic and supportive person who talks to and comforts the patient during the surgery (sometimes called "verbal anaesthesia") reduces, and often removes, the need for chemical analgesics. For apprehensive patients and those for whom a painful procedure is anticipated, sedation with a minor tranquillizer such as diazepam may be desirable. Dosage should be kept within a range that calms anxiety but does not produce sleep, as unexpected intraoperative complications are more rapidly recognized when the woman is able to report pain or other unusual symptoms during the procedure.

Anaesthesia, sedation and analgesia for elective abortion

Many of the factors described above also apply to elective abortion. In particular, verbal reassurance is essential to minimize anxiety. While most early and uncomplicated elective abortion procedures may not require analgesia, oral, intramuscular, or intravenous administration of analgesics or paracervical block can be used to reduce the pain of mechanical dilatation of the cervix or uterine curettage. Care should be taken to avoid overdose of analgesics (WHO, 1994). In addition, oral analgesics are frequently prescribed for the relief of uterine cramps in the immediate postabortion period.

The use of specialized instruments and gentle cervical dilatation with multiple osmotic dilators makes local anaesthesia, alone or in combination with mild sedation, feasible even in second-trimester D&E procedures. In this way, the patient is still responsive and can communicate with the provider. Clinics must be equipped with emergency drugs and personnel trained in their use in the event of a reaction to anaesthetic drugs.

Tissue inspection and disposal

All tissue removed in uterine evacuation must be examined visually as an integral part of the procedure. Formal tissue diagnosis by a pathology laboratory may be required in some large hospitals, though this measure is neither necessary nor economically feasible for clinics with limited resources. Visual examination, either by the naked eye or with a magnifying lens, should be carried out in all cases. The purpose of tissue inspection is:

- to verify the presence of pregnancy tissue (see pages 46–47 for management of failed evacuation);
- to ascertain completeness of evacuation in order to avoid retained tissue or continuing pregnancy;
- to identify abnormal pathological conditions such as hydatidiform mole.

A management protocol should be available for any findings that deviate from the norm to guide appropriate follow-up action and minimize complications.

Ethical and legal considerations require that procedures be established for the proper disposal of products of conception. Clinic managers must ensure that tissue disposal is accomplished in a culturally and hygienically acceptable manner and in accordance with established infection control protocols (see page 66) to avoid risk to those involved. Incineration or burial in sealed containers may be appropriate in some circumstances according to prevailing norms.

Postoperative monitoring

Immediately following any surgical procedure in abortion care, the patient's pulse, blood pressure and respiration (vital signs) should be checked. She can then be transferred to a comfortable recovery area where a trained attendant should monitor her recovery. During recovery, vital signs and pertinent symptoms should be checked periodically. Medical consultation should be sought if any of the following symptoms are observed during the postoperative period:

- significant change in vital signs;
- light-headedness, shortness of breath, or syncope;
- excessive bleeding (more than a normal menstrual flow);
- severe abdominal pain or cramps.

The patient should be discharged only when her vital signs are stable and she has fully recovered from the effects of any anaesthesia or sedation.

It has been demonstrated that women who have undergone uterine evacuation without general anaesthesia or heavy sedation, and who are not suffering from further complications requiring care, can be discharged on the same day, preferably accompanied by a friend or relative.

Discharge instructions

At discharge, women should understand what to expect during the postabortion recovery period and where care is available if it is needed. This information should be communicated verbally and, in addition, the provision of written or visual instructions is helpful. Fig. 4 gives an example of discharge instructions that may be used or adapted as appropriate. The information needed by the woman includes the following:

- signs and symptoms requiring immediate emergency care (see Table 10);
- what to do if complications occur, and sources of emergency care;
- side-effects to be expected;
- instructions for taking any medications that have been prescribed;
- aftercare, including personal cleanliness and resumption of sexual activity, resumption of menses, and family planning;

Fig. 4.   Example of printed information to accompany discharge instructions

Go to the hospital or clinic if you have:

-- severe pain
-- nausea
-- more bleeding than your
   normal menstrual flow
-- chills or fever

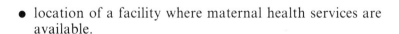

● location of a facility where maternal health services are available.

Because routine clinical follow-up is generally impractical and unnecessary following uncomplicated abortion care, routine discharge instructions must be explicit and well understood by the woman before she leaves. A return visit should be at the discretion of the woman herself and her clinician. A patient who has no symptoms requiring follow-up care should be referred to a local health care provider for continued family planning services and future gynaecological care.

Table 10. Danger signs after abortion

If any of the following symptoms are experienced by the patient after she receives emergency abortion care and is discharged from an abortion care facility, she should return for evaluation and treatment:

- fever
- chills
- muscle aches
- weakness
- abdominal pain, cramping or backache
- tenderness to pressure in the abdomen
- prolonged or heavy bleeding
- foul-smelling vaginal discharge
- delay (6 weeks or more) in resuming menstrual periods
- nausea or vomiting

Adapted from Hatcher, 1989.

Postabortion family planning

Delivery of family planning counselling and services can be challenging to managers of facilities providing emergency abortion care. Yet, in order to reduce the mortality and morbidity from unsafe abortion, it is important that providers determine whether women want to become pregnant again and address the contraceptive needs of those women who are at risk of an unwanted pregnancy. Ovulation frequently occurs by the third week after an abortion; it is clear, therefore, that women who wish to delay or avoid pregnancy should begin using contraceptives without delay.

In some facilities, having staff trained in family planning and making contraceptive methods available in the emergency care setting may be the best solution for providing postabortion family planning. In other facilities a clear protocol for family planning follow-up or an effective referral system to a family planning clinic may be a more realistic strategy. At a minimum, the woman's family planning needs should be assessed through counselling, beginning by discussing with the woman whether or not she wishes to become pregnant. Printed materials giving appropriate information can be made available (Fig. 5). Systematic follow-up and information, education and communication are necessary to ensure correct use and to support continued use whenever a family planning method is supplied.

Fig. 5.   Example of printed information on contraceptive methods

If you wish to prevent pregnancy or delay childbearing, discuss the options available with a health worker.

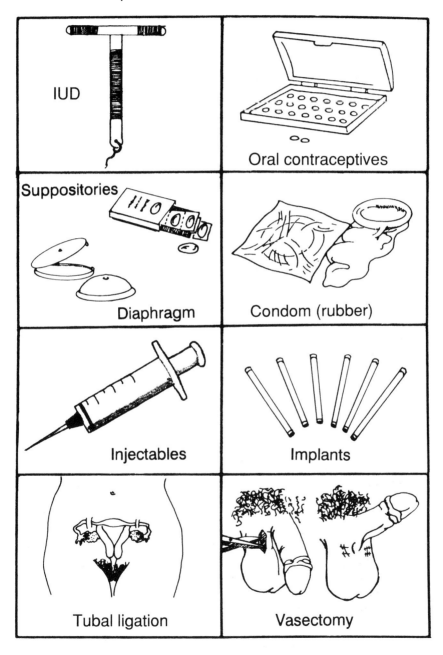

Table 11. Managerial aspects of contraceptive methods used following abortion

Method	Timing	Advantages	Remarks
Oral contraceptives	Begin use preferably on the day of the abortion or within one week.	• Highly effective if used regularly • Can be started immediately even if infection is present • Can be provided by trained non-physicians	• Require continued motivation and regular use • Resupply must be available
Intrauterine devices (IUDs)	Can be inserted immediately after first-trimester spontaneous or induced abortion, if the uterus is not infected. Expulsion rates are not higher than with interval insertions and the risk of PID is no greater. If adequate counselling and informed decision-making cannot be guaranteed, it may be best to delay insertion and provide an interim temporary method. In the second trimester, expulsion rates are lowest if insertion is delayed for six weeks, though this consideration must be balanced against the chance that an unwanted pregnancy may occur during the delay. An interim method should be used. If the uterus is infected, insertion should be delayed until the infection has resolved. An interim method should be used.	• Can be inserted by trained non-physicians • Convenient to use; not related to intercourse • Provides long-term protection • Immediate return to normal fertility following removal	• Risk of uterine perforation during insertion • May increase risk of PID and subsequent infertility for women at risk of sexually transmitted diseases • Trained provider required to discontinue use • May increase menstrual bleeding

Method	Timing	Advantages	Considerations
Implants	Insertion can take place immediately after abortion. If adequate counselling and informed decision-making cannot be guaranteed, it may be best to delay insertion and provide an interim temporary method.	• Once inserted, convenient to use • Can be administered by trained non-physicians • Provides long-term protection • Immediate return to normal fertility following removal	• May cause irregular bleeding or no bleeding; excessive bleeding may occur in rare instances • Less effective in heavier women • Trained provider required to discontinue use • Cost-effectiveness depends on long-term use • Must be replaced after 5 years to avoid a decrease in effectiveness and potential increase in risk of ectopic pregnancy
Injectables (DMPA, NET-EN)[a]	The first injection can take place immediately after abortion in the first or second trimester. If adequate counselling and informed decision-making cannot be guaranteed, it may be best to delay beginning injections and provide an interim temporary method.	• Easily administered by non-physicians • Convenient for woman; not related to intercourse	• May cause irregular bleeding; excessive bleeding may occur in rare instances • Possible delayed return to fertility • Resupply must be available • Convenient access to clinic important as regular return visits are required

Table 11 (*continued*)

Method	Timing	Advantages	Remarks
Female sterilization	It is imperative that adequate counselling and informed consent precede sterilization and this is unlikely in the emergency context. Technically, sterilization can be performed immediately after first-trimester spontaneous or elective abortion, and after treatment of abortion complications except where there is infection or severe blood loss. Sterilization after a first-trimester abortion is similar to an interval procedure. Sterilization after a second-trimester abortion is similar to a postpartum procedure.	● Permanent method	● Permanence of the method increases the importance of adequate counselling and fully informed consent; this is not likely to be possible at the time of emergency care
Male sterilization	Timing not related to abortion.	● Permanent method	● Permanence of the method increases the importance of adequate counselling and fully informed consent

Method			
Barriers not requiring fitting (condom, sponge); spermicides (suppository, foam tablets, jelly, foam)	Begin use as soon as intercourse is resumed.	• Useful as interim methods if initiation of another chosen method must be postponed • Medical supervision not required • Provide some protection against sexually transmitted diseases • Easily discontinued when pregnancy is desired	• Less effective than other methods • Require continued motivation and regular use • Resupply must be available
Fitted barriers used with spermicides (diaphragm or cervical cap with foam or jelly)	Fitting and use should be delayed until the cervix and vagina have returned to normal.	• Easily discontinued when pregnancy is desired	• Less effective than other methods • Require continued motivation and regular use • Resupply must be available
Periodic abstinence	Not recommended for immediate postabortion use. The first ovulation after an abortion will be difficult for the woman to predict and the method is unreliable until after the first postabortion menses.	• No cost	• Unreliable immediately after abortion • Alternative methods are recommended until resumption of normal cycle • Women and their partners must be motivated and have a thorough understanding of how to use the method

[a] DMPA, depot-medroxyprogesterone acetate; NET-EN, norethisterone enantate.

In the absence of severe complications or specific contraindications, oral contraceptives, intrauterine devices and sterilization are safe and effective methods for use immediately following abortion (Leonard & Ladipo, 1994), as are injectables and implants. Table 11 outlines the most important factors that managers need to know regarding the use of each method following abortion. A list of WHO publications providing more detailed information on contraception and family planning methods is provided in the additional reading section at the end of the chapter.

Adequate counselling that assists women in making free and informed choices based on information about all available methods is one of the most basic aspects of quality in family planning. Such counselling is often more difficult after emergency abortion care than during a scheduled family planning visit, for many reasons. If there is any doubt as to whether adequate counselling is possible or whether the woman is capable of making a free, informed choice at the time of treatment for abortion complications, it may be best to delay any decisions on permanent or long-term methods, or on methods requiring a provider for discontinuation. An interim method should be provided and a follow-up appointment for family planning should be arranged.

Family planning counselling and service delivery should always be available to women before their discharge following induced abortion. Studies throughout the world have consistently demonstrated that women are much more likely to use contraception after an abortion than before, and that they use more effective methods, if such methods are available.

Infection control

The essentials of infection control in abortion care are no different from those that apply to any condition involving surgical intervention. The AIDS epidemic has heightened awareness of the importance of universal precautions for strict infection control to protect health care workers and the community as well as patients. Since abortion care involves contact with blood and other body fluids, universal precautions should be understood and applied by all clinical and support staff in all facilities that provide these services. Managers must take responsibility for monitoring adherence to the most up-to-date infection control guidelines in order to protect the staff, the patients and the community. For more information on essential infection control practices, see Annex 1 or the references listed in the additional reading section at the end of the chapter. Since information on infection control is continually being updated, it is important to obtain the most recent publications from authoritative sources. The essential elements for infection control at all levels of abortion care are:

- thorough handwashing and use of protective gloves;
- a clean, well ventilated facility;
- an adequate supply of clean water;
- adequate decontamination procedures for all instruments immediately after each use;
- meticulous attention to sterilization and disinfection of equipment and supplies;
- strict asepsis during operative procedures;
- use of barrier precautions to protect clinical and support staff whenever they may come into contact with blood and other body fluids; appropriate barriers may include gloves, masks, waterproof gowns, and protective eyewear if available;
- precautions against accidental cuts and needle-stick accidents among staff;
- careful handling of all wastes, dirty linen and equipment;
- appropriate disposal of all blood and tissue as well as contaminated materials;
- immediate handwashing if contaminated with blood or other body fluids, and always upon removal of gloves.

It is important to ensure that any instrument or part of an instrument to be inserted through the cervical canal does not touch any non-sterile object or surface prior to insertion.

When plastic cannulae and vacuum aspiration syringes are used, it is essential that they are properly cleaned and maintained. Before reuse, cannulae need to be sterilized or disinfected at high level. Most plastic cannulae cannot be autoclaved; however, some can be boiled. If boiling is not possible, chemical disinfection following established protocols for high-level disinfection may be used.[1] Vacuum aspiration syringes must be clean and disinfected, but it is not necessary to sterilize them.

Infection control merits special attention in the management of quality assurance at all clinical levels (see Annex 1). Frequent

---

[1] High-level disinfection is the destruction of all microbes, but not necessarily spores present in large numbers (WHO, 1989).

supervision of infection control practices, spot checks of equipment sterilization and disinfection, careful monitoring of techniques and solutions to determine the adequacy of sterilization and disinfection, routine maintenance of autoclaves, sterilizers, and chemical disinfection equipment, and periodic medical audits of infection rates are required to ensure maximum safety. Moreover, since infection control recommendations are subject to change as new information becomes available, managers should provide all health care workers with appropriate in-service education regarding current infection control practices and safety precautions (Centers for Disease Control, 1991).

Management of rhesus-negative abortion patients

Sensitization to the rhesus (Rh) factor can occur during an interrupted pregnancy, although the risk is low in the early weeks of gestation. In populations where significant numbers of women are Rh-negative, clinics that have the resources for Rh testing and administration of Rh immune globulin should provide this service. The injection can be given at the time of treatment or immediately after an induced abortion but should be given in all cases within 72 hours to prevent isoimmunization.

Laboratory requirements

Limited resources at some health service levels often preclude the use of many laboratory tests in emergency abortion care. Determination of haemoglobin or haematocrit (erythrocyte volume fraction) to detect anaemia is advisable for all women undergoing uterine evacuation. As these tests may not be available at some centres, an empirical assessment of blood loss can and should be made rather than risking lives by postponing care. If a woman is anaemic and in need of blood or other fluid replacement and if these services are not available at her first point of contact with the health system, she should be referred to a higher level of service for treatment as quickly as possible.

All services at the first referral level should have the capacity to undertake blood crossmatching and transfusions. Supplies of packed blood cells and blood substitutes should also be available.

Laboratory tests that are highly desirable, though not essential, for emergency abortion care are noted below:

● pregnancy tests;
● bacterial smears or cultures for detection of sexually transmitted diseases and other infections of the genital tract;

- Papanicolaou smears for cervical cancer screening.

Where circumstances permit, generally at the secondary or tertiary levels, the tests and facilities listed below may be available:

- tests for hepatitis, human immunodeficiency virus (HIV) and syphilis;
- hormone assays for management and follow-up of certain high-risk conditions, such as trophoblastic disease and ectopic pregnancy;
- testing for diagnosis of congenital or genetic disorders;
- imaging equipment, preferably ultrasound, to assist in the accurate determination of gestational age, diagnosis of extrauterine pregnancy, and to provide visual guidance to minimize the risks of abortion procedures in late pregnancy and in abnormally shaped or positioned uteri.

References

CENTERS FOR DISEASE CONTROL (1991) Recommendations for preventing transmission of human immunodeficiency virus and hepatitis B virus to patients during exposure-prone invasive procedures. *Morbidity and mortality weekly report*, **40**(RR-8): 1–9.

DARNEY PD, ed. (1987) *Handbook of office & ambulatory gynecologic surgery*. Oradell, New Jersey, Medical Economics Books.

DOBSON MB (1988) *Anaesthesia at the district hospital*. Geneva, World Health Organization.

HATCHER RA (1989) *Contraceptive technology: international edition*. Atlanta, Printed Matter, Inc.

KING M, ed. (1986) *Primary anaesthesia*. Oxford, Oxford University Press.

LEONARD AH, LADIPO OA (1994) Post-abortion family planning: factors in individual choice of contraceptive methods. *Advances in abortion care*, **4**(2): 1–4.

LISKIN LS (1980) Complications of abortion in developing countries. *Population reports*, Series F, No. 7.

MARX GF ET AL. (1978) Postpartum uterine pressures under halothane or enflurane anesthesia. *Obstetrics and gynecology*, **51**(6): 695–698.

NASSER J (1989) Commentary on pain management during abortion from a Latin American physician's perspective. In: Rosenfield A et al., eds. Women's health in the Third World: the impact of unwanted pregnancy. *International journal of gynecology and obstetrics*, Suppl. 3: 141–143.

SAI FT, NASSIM J (1989) The need for a reproductive health approach. In: Rosenfield A et al., eds. Women's health in the Third World: the impact of unwanted pregnancy. *International journal of gynecology and obstetrics*, Suppl. 3: 103–113.

WHO (1989) *Guidelines on sterilization and disinfection methods effective against human immunodeficiency virus (HIV)*, 2nd ed. Geneva, World Health Organization (WHO AIDS Series No. 2).

WHO (1994) *Clinical management of abortion complications.* Geneva, World Health Organization (unpublished document WHO/FHE/MSM/94.1).

Additional reading

WHO publications and documents on contraception and family planning

Barrier contraceptives and spermicides: their role in family planning care. 1987.

Contraceptive method mix. Guidelines for policy and service delivery. 1994.

Female sterilization: a guide to provision of services. 1992.

Injectable contraceptives: their role in family planning care. 1990.

Mechanism of action, safety and efficacy of intrauterine devices. Report of a WHO Scientific Group, 1987 (WHO Technical Report Series, No. 753).

Natural family planning: a guide to provision of services. 1988.

Norplant contraceptive subdermal implants: managerial and technical guidelines (provisional version). 1990 (unpublished document WHO/MCH/89.17).

Oral contraceptives: technical and safety aspects. 1982 (WHO Offset Publication No. 64).

Technical and managerial guidelines for vasectomy services. 1988.

Publications and documents on infection control

ANGLE M ET AL. *Sterilization, disinfection, decontamination and cleaning of FP/MCH clinic equipment.* Chapel Hill, University of North Carolina, Program for International Training in Health, 1989 (INTRAH training information packet).

CENTERS FOR DISEASE CONTROL. Guidelines for prevention of transmission of human immunodeficiency virus and hepatitis B virus to health-care and public-safety workers. *Morbidity and mortality weekly report* **38**(S-6): 3–37 (1989).

WORLD HEALTH ORGANIZATION. *AIDS prevention: guidelines for MCH/FP programme managers. I. AIDS and family planning.* Geneva, 1990 (unpublished document WHO/MCH/GPA/90.1).

WORLD HEALTH ORGANIZATION. *AIDS prevention: guidelines for MCH/FP programme managers. II. AIDS and maternal and child health.* Geneva, 1990 (unpublished document WHO/MCH/GPA/90.2).

WORLD HEALTH ORGANIZATION. *Guidelines for nursing management of people infected with human immunodeficiency virus (HIV).* Geneva, 1988 (WHO AIDS Series No. 3).

Chapter 8

INFORMATION AND COUNSELLING FOR THE PATIENT

Counselling ... implies more than simply offering information and an expert professional opinion ... [it] also entails *listening* to [each person's] special, individual needs and circumstances. It allows the person concerned to take an active rather than a passive role in the decision-making process. In particular, it goes beyond mere questions of "fact" and includes a discussion and exploration of feelings and relationships (Kleinman, 1988).

Needs for medical information

As in any medical procedure, women who are undergoing abortion or who are being treated for complications of abortion need information regarding their personal situation. The timing and content will vary depending on the woman's condition and her immediate physical needs. Managers should ensure that the information needed by the woman and her family is provided in a supportive, non-judgemental, and confidential manner.

Emergency abortion care

Health care workers must be trained and prepared to discuss confidentially the issues below with each woman receiving emergency abortion care and, as the woman wishes or as necessary, with whoever accompanies her.

The woman's health status

— Overall physical condition
— Results of the physical and pelvic examination
— Laboratory findings

The proposed treatment plan

— Time-frame for treatment
— Need for referral and transport to another facility or department, as required

— Procedures to be used and the risks and benefits of each

— Consent for treatment by the woman or, if she is unable, a family member or other responsible adult

Postoperative care (see page 58)

— Anticipated postoperative discomfort and how to ease it

— Symptoms of postoperative complications indicating the need for medical attention and how such attention can be obtained

— When and where to go for any scheduled follow-up care and family planning

— Ways that the partner and family can help ensure a speedy recovery

— Timing of any subsequent pregnancy and contraceptive options

Elective abortion

Women seeking an elective abortion should be given all the information listed above and in addition, should be told about the following:

— requirements and procedures for obtaining the abortion;

— risks, benefits, and efficacy of alternative abortion techniques, if more than one is available.

Consent for treatment

Consent for treatment refers to the process by which a patient learns about a procedure and then, on the basis of complete and accurate information, makes a free, informed choice to undergo the procedure. In some jurisdictions, written consent may be required for all operative procedures, including those performed for emergency treatment of abortion complications. However, under no circumstances should consent requirements delay or interfere with providing emergency treatment to save a woman's life. Informed consent should be an element of all elective abortion services.

The health care worker obtaining the woman's consent for treatment should follow these steps:

● Determine whether the woman is capable of listening to and understanding medical explanations. If she is not, consent for treatment should be discussed instead with the woman's representative.

- Explain in detail, in a non-threatening manner and in language the woman can understand, the procedure or procedures to be performed, including risks, benefits, likelihood of success, and alternatives.

- Allow time for and encourage the woman to ask questions and discuss the procedures.

- Ask the woman to give consent for treatment. If she is unable to do so owing to her condition, her representative may give consent on her behalf.

Counselling

Counselling—face-to-face communication in which a counsellor assists the woman in making her own decisions and acting on them—must be a part of all abortion care. Whenever possible, counselling should precede treatment. Ideally, the same counsellor should provide support before, during, and after treatment; however, this is often difficult in a health care facility with limited staff and high caseloads. Nevertheless, a supportive and caring staff can do much to meet the psychological and emotional needs of women seeking emergency abortion care or elective abortion.

Counselling in abortion care can be provided by a variety of staff members, including nurses, midwives, physicians, social workers or nurse aides. Volunteers have been used successfully in some situations. A professional counsellor is not necessary; however, training in counselling techniques should be provided for any staff functioning as counsellors.

Staff who provide counselling must be non-judgemental, extremely sensitive to and respectful of the woman's emotions and feelings, in order to adapt the session to the woman's specific needs. Counsellors should be knowledgeable, well-trained, and able to give accurate information. Counselling staff must always be aware of the need for privacy, confidentiality, and, in some cases, anonymity (Edmunds, 1987). Critical elements of all good counselling include the ability of the counsellor to elicit and listen to a woman's needs, concerns and questions, and to inform, educate and reassure using language and terms that the woman understands (Kleinman, 1988). It is also useful to augment verbal explanations with written and pictorial materials to reinforce what has been said in the counselling session (Fig. 6).

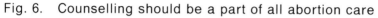

Fig. 6.   Counselling should be a part of all abortion care

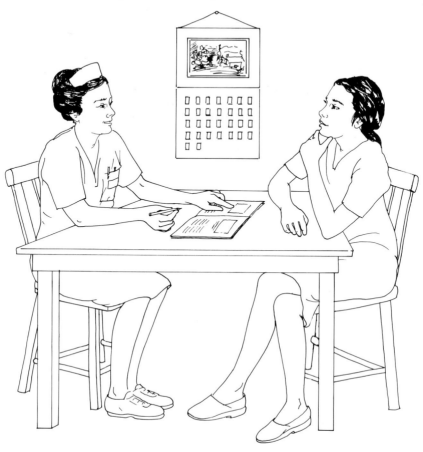

Supportive counselling

Supportive counselling is the provision of psychosocial support. Women who have had an abortion may need help in handling the emotional and psychological response to the experience. Some women may be worried or anxious about how they will be treated by family, friends and the community after their recovery. Others may have concerns about the care of their children and other family members during their absence for treatment.

It is important that women receiving emergency care or elective abortion have an opportunity to discuss their health, feelings, and personal situation with a knowledgeable, sensitive, non-judgemental counsellor. Counsellors must refrain from imposing their views and beliefs on the women they counsel and must hold all information in confidence. Counsellors should be able to help women clarify their feelings as well as how they will deal with these feelings when they return home.

For certain women, supportive counselling when receiving abortion care is especially important and continued counselling after discharge may be beneficial. If the facility providing abortion care does not have sufficient staff or staff with adequate skills to provide continued counselling, the women should be referred to a facility where counselling is available. Women for whom special attention to supportive counselling may be required include:

- adolescents and very young women, regardless of marital status;

- women with obvious signs of distress or a history of emotional problems;

- women suffering from complications of abortion;

- women undergoing elective abortion on medical grounds;

- women having a late elective abortion;

- women aborting a pregnancy resulting from rape or incest;

- women infected with HIV (see page 29);

- women with marital, family or socioeconomic problems;

- women who have experienced unwanted pregnancy resulting from contraceptive failure.

Family planning counselling

Induced abortion, whether it occurs in an unsafe setting or in accordance with legal requirements, almost always indicates a desire to avoid or postpone childbearing. For this reason, it is important that all facilities, whether providing emergency care or elective abortion, offer family planning counselling and services. (See page 60 and Table 11 for more information on post-abortion family planning. References on family planning are listed on page 70.) If it is impossible to provide family planning services in conjunction with abortion care, women should be counselled and referred to a nearby family planning service delivery point.

The provision of emergency abortion care or elective abortion procedures must not be made conditional on the acceptance of family planning in general, or of a specific method of contraception. Women need information on a wide range of contraceptive methods in order to make their own selection, in consultation with clinic staff. Managers can ensure that coercion is not being used in method selection by monitoring trends in contraceptive distribution to women after abortion.

References

EDMUNDS M ET AL. (1987) *Client-responsive family planning: a handbook for providers.* Watertown, MA, Pathfinder Fund.

KLEINMAN RL, ed. (1988) *Family planning handbook for doctors*, 6th ed. London, International Planned Parenthood Federation.

Chapter 9

FACILITIES AND EQUIPMENT

> Except in the case of severe complications, most emergency abortion care can be provided in existing facilities with little specialized equipment.

It is the responsibility of managers to see that facilities and equipment are adequate for provision of the safest possible abortion care at the lowest feasible level in the health care system. In most cases, minor adaptations of existing facilities, changes in patient flow or the acquisition of minimal new equipment can improve the safety and efficiency of abortion care and allow for expanded service provision. Such minor adaptations can greatly increase the number of service delivery points available for emergency abortion care.

Facilities for emergency abortion care

During the first trimester of pregnancy, emergency care can be provided for uncomplicated cases at the primary or first referral level, since sophisticated medical equipment, specialized staff, and operating rooms are usually not required. Care can usually be provided within the gynaecology unit or in the emergency room on an outpatient basis. Uterine evacuation by vacuum aspiration can be carried out by trained staff in a simple treatment room and the woman can usually be discharged after a short recovery period and after she has received and understood discharge instructions. Dilatation and curettage can also be performed, though this usually requires a more specialized facility.

Care for serious complications and in the later stages of pregnancy should be provided in a setting with more specialized facilities and personnel. Hospitalization is often required; however, many services deliver emergency care for uncomplicated abortion in late gestation on an outpatient basis. A full-scale operating room is not required, unless laparotomy is anticipated or general anaesthesia is needed.

Every effort should be made to provide clinical care and counselling in a private environment. In some facilities, a separate

Table 12. Equipment and facilities for abortion care

Staff	Activities	Facilities	Equipment/drugs
A. Community level			
The level of responsibility varies from country to country depending on the primary health care programme. Good communications between community health workers and the primary level are essential.			
Community health workers with basic health training including:	Recognition of abortion and complications	There are usually no formal health care facilities at this level	No equipment or drugs are required for these activities. A few drugs (e.g., antimalarials) may be available.
• traditional birth attendants (TBAs)	Timely referral to the formal health care system		
• traditional healers	Health education regarding unsafe abortion		Good communication channels with the primary care level are essential.
• community residents			
			Health education materials (handouts, charts, etc.) are helpful.
	Family planning information, education and services		Counselling materials (leaflets, posters, etc.) are helpful.
			Some contraceptives (e.g. condoms, oral contraceptives, spermicides) may be provided.

B. Primary level

The activities will depend on the skills available. Existing facilities are usually adequate. Rearrangement of facilities and updating of equipment may be all that is required to improve the abortion care provided. Some facilities may already have equipment for uterine evacuation on hand but some may need to purchase it. Protocols and standing arrangements for transport to higher levels are necessary. If an ambulance is available, it must be kept in a serviceable state. If no ambulance is available, standing arrangements for transport should be made with other sectors. It is important to have a reliable system of communication with the other levels of care.

Staff	Services/activities	Facilities	Equipment
Auxiliary health workers including: • health assistants • aides • dispensers/dressers Nurses Some primary level facilities may have the following staff available: • trained midwives • medical residents • general practitioners	All those listed for the community level plus: Simple physical and pelvic examination Diagnosis of stages of abortion Resuscitation and preparation for treatment or transfer (if needed) including: • management of the airway and respiration • control of bleeding • pain control • haematocrit and haemoglobin determination Referral Postabortion family planning counselling and services *If trained staff and appropriate equipment are available, the following additional activities can be performed:* • Initiation of essential treatment, including antibiotic therapy, intravenous fluid replacement, and oxytocics • Uterine evacuation (first trimester) • Pain control including paracervical block, simple analgesia and sedation	Outpatient treatment room or area Side laboratory Family planning area or clinic Separate room or private corner of treatment room	Examination couches Gloves, protective clothing Light sources Vaginal specula Soap, disinfectants Standard emergency resuscitation kit (see Annex 3A) Transport vehicle or standing arrangements for transport Essential drugs (see Annex 3C) Side laboratory equipment (see Annex 3G) Wide range of contraceptives including IUD insertion kit Broad-spectrum antibiotics Uterine evacuation kits (vacuum aspiration or D&C) (see Annex 2B) Sterilization equipment or disinfectant solutions Agent for local anaesthesia Sedatives Analgesics Needles and syringes

Table 12 (continued)

Staff	Activities	Facilities	Equipment/drugs
C. First referral level			
Most facilities and equipment needed for treatment of abortion complications will already be available in a district hospital for general emergencies and essential obstetric functions. Some expansion and additional equipment may be necessary. Supply logistics and maintenance procedures may need to be strengthened. A serviceable ambulance should be on hand or other transport arrangements made. Radio or telephone contact with the tertiary and primary levels is important as is coordination and collaboration with maternal and child health activities at the community level.			
All those listed for the primary level plus:	All those listed for the primary level plus:	Treatment room in outpatient area or gynaecology ward and recovery area	Sufficient quantity of uterine evacuation equipment for projected caseload (see Annex 2C, D and E)
Trained midwives	Uterine evacuation for first and second trimester		Essential drugs for the first referral level (see Annex 2C)
Medical residents	Treatment of most abortion complications	Laboratory	Laboratory equipment and reagents for microscopy, culture and basic haematology (see Annex 2G)
General practitioners	Blood crossmatching and transfusion	Surgical theatre	Blood or blood substitutes
Specialists, including a physician with training in obstetrics/gynaecology may sometimes be available	Local and general anaesthesia		Equipment for blood collection, transfusion and storage (see Annex 2G)
	Laparotomy and indicated surgery, including surgery for ectopic pregnancy if skilled staff are available		Anaesthetic equipment
	Pregnancy testing		Standard laparotomy set (see Annex 2F)
	Diagnosis and referral of severe complications such as septicaemia, peritonitis or renal failure		Pregnancy tests
			Ambulance
			Full range of contraceptives

D. Secondary and tertiary levels

Most of the facilities and equipment are available. Rearrangement of patient flow or expansion of facilities may improve services. Additional equipment is likely to include vacuum aspiration equipment.

All of those listed for the first referral level plus:	All of those listed for the first referral level plus:	Treatment room in outpatient or inpatient gynaecological areas	All of those listed for the first referral level plus:
Specialists in obstetrics, gynaecology and allied specialities	Uterine evacuation for all abortions	24-hour access to surgical theatre (may include a specific gynaecological emergency theatre)	More elaborate anaesthetic and intensive care equipment
	Treatment of severe complications (for example, bowel injury, tetanus, renal failure, gas gangrene, severe sepsis, septic shock, coagulopathy) including: ● diagnostic X-ray ● ultrasonography ● laparoscopy ● laparotomy including hysterectomy	More complete laboratory facilities	X-ray equipment
		Intensive care facilities	Sorography equipment
		Shielded X-ray room	Laparoscope
		Blood bank	

room may be available for treatment or for counselling and recovery, but if not, privacy can be ensured by placing screens around a bed, cot, or couch in a gynaecology ward or emergency room.

Table 12 lists the equipment and facilities needed for abortion care at each level of the health care system, based on the usual staffing pattern and the elements of care that can be provided at each level.

Facilities for elective abortion

Elective abortions may be delivered within an integrated gynaecology ward, in a free-standing facility or in a dedicated abortion unit of a health facility. During the first trimester, these services can generally be provided on an outpatient basis. Later procedures should be handled in well-equipped settings with specially trained staff.

If possible, elective abortion should not be provided at the same time and place or by the same staff as antenatal clinics or well baby clinics, or next to obstetric units and nurseries, or in similar settings that might create emotional difficulties for both patients and staff and make it difficult for the staff to deal with what could be perceived as conflicting values.

Outpatient care

In most cases, emergency abortion care and elective abortion can and should be delivered in an outpatient setting with minimal use of anaesthesia. Care should be delivered at the lowest level of the health system that can safely deliver it. Generally, appropriately trained staff and adequate equipment can be made available at the primary or first referral level. Emergency care must be available 24 hours a day. Shifting care out of operating theatres and into treatment rooms or ambulatory care centres at the primary and first referral levels is a major benefit for any hospital or clinic and for the women they serve. Some of the benefits of offering abortion care at lower levels of the health system on an outpatient basis are:

- improved access to services by providing abortion care as an outpatient service and treating some women—who would otherwise be referred—at lower level facilities;
- reduced crowding and delay in treatment as a result of more efficient use of hospital beds and operating room facilities;

- more timely treatment, since transportation and waiting time required for referral or inpatient admission procedures are eliminated;
- increased availability of operating theatre facilities and staff for other procedures;
- fewer patients who must be referred to the secondary and tertiary levels, allowing those centres to focus on care requiring the extra resources available only at the higher levels of the health care system.

Caseload considerations

In planning for emergency or elective abortion care, it is important to know the current and projected abortion caseloads. The current caseload can be quantified by reviewing hospital and clinic records. Problems stemming from a high caseload may be obvious to the manager. For example, women waiting for treatment may be filling the hallways, there may be a lengthy wait for treatment, or the bed occupancy rate may be too high. This congestion could indicate a particularly high caseload or poor patient flow (see below).

Managers should monitor the current caseload frequently and remain alert to developments that could affect the projected caseload. Some of the factors that cause the caseload to fluctuate include changes in access to contraception, changes in population distribution, efforts to encourage particular groups such as adolescents to seek care, changes in the structure of the health system or the referral network, reassignment of staff, construction of additional health care facilities in the community, introduction of similar services in the same catchment area, or a change in the abortion laws.

Patient flow

Effective systems for managing the flow of patients through a facility ensure that, regardless of fluctuations in caseload, women receive care in a logical sequence and without unnecessary delay. Managers can often improve the quality of care significantly by organizing existing resources more efficiently. Three critical questions that managers can examine to improve patient flow are:

- What activities must be carried out in a particular area, and in what order?
- Where and why does congestion occur?

- How could use of space and personnel be modified to increase the efficiency of activities and better serve the patients?

Examples of ways to make patient flow more efficient include: performing uterine evacuation in the casualty ward rather than referring cases to the gynaecology ward; treating most cases on an outpatient basis; and using treatment rooms rather than operating theatres.

Use of space and staff in a way that fosters smooth patient flow and minimizes delays may be difficult in a casualty ward setting. Presentation of patients for emergency abortion care is unpredictable, so managers must plan for fluctuations in caseload and maintain service delivery 24 hours a day. Elective abortion care may be established within fixed hours and is more predictable.

Equipment and drugs for emergency and elective abortion care

Good quality abortion care does not require extensive specialized equipment and drugs. Managers must be concerned with the logistics of obtaining the necessary equipment and supplies, seeing that they are available when and where services are delivered, and supervising their maintenance. They must consider the initial investment for equipment, the recurring cost of disposable supplies, and the cost savings of preventing serious complications. Some important considerations regarding the purchase, supply, and maintenance of equipment are listed below.

- What is the current status of abortion care services and what material resources exist?
- What equipment and supplies are needed?
- What quantity of equipment and supplies will be needed?
- What are the inventory control issues?
- What policies and procedures are needed to manage the logistics of obtaining and maintaining equipment?

These questions and some managerial responses to each are discussed below.

Current status and existing resources for abortion care

The equipment needs for treatment of uncomplicated incomplete abortion are not elaborate and most of the items will be part of the existing inventory of primary and first referral level facilities. Likewise, the equipment needed for treatment of serious complications should be available at institutions that provide general or gynaecological surgery.

In some cases managers may wish to adapt current facilities or procedures to deliver more efficient or broader abortion-related care, for example, by establishing an outpatient treatment room. In this context, additional equipment and supplies may be required to create new treatment areas. In other cases the addition of only a few simple pieces of equipment, such as a light or examining table, may be needed.

In any setting, particular care must be taken to ensure that the procedure area is well stocked with supplies in order to avoid interruptions in care.

Equipment and supplies needed

The medical equipment and supplies needed will depend largely on the type of procedures to be offered at the facility. Table 12 lists the equipment and drug requirements for abortion care at each level of the health care system. Detailed lists of equipment and supply needs are given in Annex 2. All facilities must have supplies for resuscitation as well as drugs to control haemorrhage readily available (see Annex 2A). Supplies must be adequate to meet emergency needs and should be replenished promptly when used.

Where there is a choice, the costs and benefits of disposable supplies (those discarded after a single use) and non-disposable items (those processed for reuse) must be carefully weighed. Disposable supplies are generally more expensive. Since they must be reordered regularly, these supplies are also subject to shortages in stock and problems with shipment. Furthermore, disposal of such supplies must be in accordance with standard infection control measures (see Annex 1). When non-disposable supplies and equipment are used, staff must be trained in how to clean and maintain them properly and supervised regularly in these tasks. Costs will be incurred in purchasing the reagents needed for sterilization and disinfection. Non-disposable supplies will require particular diligence in the adherence to routine infection control protocols (see Annex 1) and may be more expensive initially.

Some aspects of abortion care, such as sterilizing and disinfecting instruments or conducting laboratory tests, may be carried out centrally in larger service facilities at the first referral level and above. In these cases, managers may not need to make provisions for equipment and supplies related to these activities.

The type of equipment used may also be influenced by such factors as the availability and dependability of an electricity supply. If electricity is available but not dependable and electric equipment is to be used, a standby generator or manual back-up equipment must be purchased and maintained in good working order. In many cases, non-electric equipment may be preferable for other reasons. The complexity of equipment and the availability of replacement parts and repair services must also be considered when determining the type of equipment to be purchased.

Quantity of equipment and supplies needed

Estimates of the projected caseload and regular monitoring of services are needed to determine the quantity of equipment and supplies required (see page 83 and Chapters 4 and 12). An adequate stock of equipment must be on hand in the unit during all hours when services are provided. If equipment and instruments are sterilized centrally rather than within the unit where they are used, it is especially important to have an adequate supply and to make sure that sterilized equipment is available in the treatment area whenever it is needed.

Inventory control and maintenance

Inventory control and maintenance of equipment are essential to ensure that services will not be disrupted because equipment is missing or broken or supplies are out of stock. In planning a system for inventory control and maintenance, some issues that managers must plan for are:

● the quantity and types of equipment and supplies to be kept in stock;

● adequate storage facilities (for example, facilities that are refrigerated, pest-free, ventilated, or moisture-free, as required for each item);

● monitoring of stock levels;

● re-ordering of stock;

● security of stock;

● rotation of stock on a first in, first out basis, i.e., the oldest items or those purchased earliest should be used first;

- procedure for supply within the institution for all sites of service delivery (for example, there may be procedure rooms in both the casualty ward and the gynaecology ward);
- procedure for supply between facilities for centrally controlled systems;
- routine maintenance of equipment;
- repair of equipment;
- monitoring of equipment maintenance and supply logistics.

The location (urban or rural) of the abortion care facility influences both the ready availability of supplies and equipment and the planning time-frame required for ordering and receiving disposable items. For instance, if a hospital is a two-day journey from the nearest provider of essential supplies and the communications and transportation are unreliable, the manager will need to place an order several weeks before the supplies are expected to be needed to be assured of timely delivery. Systems must be developed to monitor the inventory of supplies in order to avoid shortages.

Managers should also consider the issues involved in the delivery system that will be used for future supplies. A staff member should be responsible for keeping records of items ordered and received from an outside agency or individual. If supplies must be obtained in person, a staff member should be made responsible and provided with transportation and the capability to pay for supplies.

Attention should be given to the security of supplies and the appropriateness of storage facilities. For example, drug expiry dates must be checked and proper temperature and humidity maintained for storage of sensitive drugs and other supplies. Equipment should be securely stored to prevent theft.

Programme managers must ensure that staff are designated to be responsible for all the tasks listed above. Special training may be needed in the maintenance and repair of surgical and other mechanical equipment. In such cases, the trainees should be monitored regularly to ensure that the skills learned are being applied (see page 104).

Policies and procedures

Managers of abortion care services must ensure that policies and procedures for storage and handling of all medical equipment and supplies are known and followed. Each institution should develop written protocols for routine maintenance of equipment and criteria for monitoring and evaluating each of the following aspects:

- an approved list of medical supplies that may be ordered;
- inventory control, including records of inventory received, distributed, or discarded;
- rotation of supplies using the first in, first out system (this is especially important for any material bearing expiry dates);
- procedures for storage and handling, security, and safe discarding of all disposable (single-use) items, such as needles and syringes;
- preventive maintenance;
- plans for continued operation in the event of equipment breakdown or malfunction;
- cleaning, sterilization and dating of equipment and supplies;
- wrapping and storage instructions for sterilized equipment and instruments;
- management of contaminated equipment and supplies.

Chapter 10

PERSONNEL: TASKS, TRAINING AND SUPERVISION

In abortion care, as in other aspects of health care, the manager's role is to see that personnel are competent, available and adequately supervised in delivery of all services required.

At the national level, managers must look at ways of ensuring that all levels of the health care system have adequate staff who have received appropriate training to perform the services required of them. Service managers at facilities must be concerned with assigning tasks to appropriate staff, supervising all categories of workers, planning regular in-service training, scheduling and handling staff rotation, and monitoring performance to maintain the highest possible standards of competence among staff members.

Tasks in abortion care

The starting point for facility managers in personnel planning is a review of the tasks that must be done and the skills of the staff available to perform those tasks. Staff can then be assigned to carry out tasks according to their training and competence, and the needs of the facility. In general, each task should be carried out by the least specialized person who has been trained to perform it competently. The tasks assigned to particular categories of health care workers vary from area to area.

Experience has shown that, in the face of limited professional staff and resources, many of the tasks traditionally performed by specialized medical staff can be safely performed by well-trained auxiliary health workers. For this reason, in discussing personnel, these guidelines specify tasks rather than job titles. The following service-related tasks must be assigned to staff in delivering both emergency abortion care and elective abortion, where available:

- emergency resuscitation and preparation for referral and transport, if necessary;

- diagnosis and determination of a treatment plan including history, medical examination, and determining the size of the uterus and status of the pregnancy;
- surgical and medical management including uterine evacuation and treatment of complications;
- provision of information and health education;
- counselling;
- laboratory tests and tissue examination;
- preoperative and postoperative monitoring and care;
- record-keeping and analysis of information for internal management purposes;
- infection control;
- clinical supervision.

Managerial tasks in the provision of abortion care are noted in the introduction to Chapter 4 and discussed throughout these guidelines.

Training

The nature of abortion care changes from time to time with the introduction of new techniques or as a result of research findings. Managers must be attuned to the need for basic training of all health care workers as well as the need to update knowledge and maintain or refresh skills in response to these changes.

Formal training

Formal education includes all the classes and training received in school, residencies, and internships, usually before a person begins working independently. As mentioned in previous chapters, it is imperative that all health care workers (physicians, midwives, social workers, nurses, emergency medical technicians, etc.) who have contact with women of reproductive age are knowledgeable about abortion care. These persons need to receive training, as part of their formal education, that is relevant to their role in providing emergency abortion care. Policy-makers and managers at the national level should ensure that abortion issues are included in the curricula for training all health care personnel. The most important types of information are outlined below.

Basic information that should be included in the curricula for all health care personnel

● The role of abortion in maternal mortality and morbidity.

● Abortion care norms and regulations for the country.

● The response of the health care system to the need for emergency abortion care.

● How to reduce the incidence of unsafe abortion, i.e. information on all available methods of contraception.

Additional knowledge and skills for those who provide clinical services

● Basic anatomy and physiology of the female reproductive system.

● Evolution of pregnancy and stages of abortion.

● Signs and symptoms of stages and complications of abortion.

● Ability to perform a general physical examination.

● Ability to conduct a basic pelvic examination, including assessment of uterine size.

● Protocols for emergency abortion care.

● All available methods of uterine evacuation (see Chapter 6).

● Management of haemorrhage, infection, and injury to the genital tract and internal organs (see page 43).

● Principles and practice of asepsis.

● Use of anaesthesia and analgesia (see page 55).

● Infection control practices (see page 66).

● Identification of pregnancy tissue (see page 57).

● Counselling and psychological support of patients (see page 73).

● Family planning counselling, contraceptive methods, and provision of family planning services (see pages 60 and 75).

In-service training

In-service training (also known as continuing education or refresher training) includes any training that health care workers receive after their formal education, which serves to update, maintain, or teach skills for the provision of health care (Abbatt & Mejia, 1988). Such training activities can have a rapid and direct effect on improving the quality of care, such as lowering complication rates (see Chapter 12). In-service training should be a regular activity at any health care facility. There are various formats for in-service training, including workshops at the facility or in a central location, regular classes to coincide with staff rotation patterns, and seminars given by local or national experts. In-service training is essential to maintain skills learned in formal training, to practise or improve counselling skills, to introduce or improve medical techniques, to transfer skills to less specialized health care workers, to spread information about changes in protocols, and to ensure that the level of competence remains high when staff rotations occur.

Monitoring and supervision activities should prompt managers to conduct in-service training. For example, a medical review may determine that a certain antibiotic has been particularly effective in managing sepsis and information on its use should be communicated to all clinicians, or a survey of patient attitudes and knowledge may prompt a seminar to improve communication skills.

Some of the in-service training activities that might be needed in abortion care services are:

- a workshop for nurses on procedures for sterilizing and disinfecting equipment;
- a seminar to train health care workers in new techniques for uterine evacuation;
- a regional meeting to introduce new protocols for referral of patients from primary to first referral level;
- a conference to disseminate information about changes in legal restrictions on elective abortion;
- a lecture by a visiting expert on the use of newly available antibiotics;
- a self-instructional course on infection control practices in obstetrics and gynaecology;
- a workshop on counselling techniques.

It is important that all health care workers benefit from training activities. For example, if nursing supervisors attend a seminar on psychosocial support of patients in abortion care, they should systematically pass on the new information and skills to the nurses they supervise. If training activities are held during the day, it is essential that a system be established to ensure that workers on duty at night are trained as well. As staff rotations occur, training activities should be repeated. If community health workers and traditional healers are involved in providing information and education about the dangers of unsafe abortion practices, they may also need periodic in-service training. While reaching this group may be difficult, it is essential to include them in training to the extent possible.

Competency-based training

Training programmes should be competency-based, that is, designed to develop competence in designated tasks. Learning objectives should specify what the participants should be able to do after training. It is important to have a clear understanding of the desired competence that training is intended to bring about in order to determine whether the training is successful. All lectures, activities, educational materials and evaluation should relate to the objectives. Examples of learning objectives for providers of vacuum aspiration are that they should be able to:

- perform vacuum aspiration to treat incomplete abortion or terminate a pregnancy in accordance with local restrictions and hospital standards;
- recognize contraindications and provide appropriate management and referral;
- provide appropriate family planning counselling and services or referral for those services;
- maintain and sterilize or disinfect vacuum aspiration equipment.

An example of a training curriculum outline for one method of uterine evacuation is presented in Annex 3A. It should be adapted as appropriate to meet the training needs of individual facilities.

Evaluation of training

In order to check that training efforts have been successful, trainees should be evaluated in relation to the learning objectives. The evaluation may take many forms. For example, knowledge can be evaluated by written tests before and after training, through interviews, or by observing trainees' performance on the job. Clinical skills should be evaluated by direct observation by a skilled clinician and, ideally, by using a written checklist of criteria dealing with key points (see Annex 3B). A similar evaluation technique can be used to assess counselling skills (see Annex 3C). Evaluators should provide direct feedback to learners, including recommendations on what they can do to improve their skills. In most situations, follow-up evaluations should be conducted several weeks or months after completion of training. The same process used for evaluation at the end of a course is appropriate for follow-up evaluation.

Staff supervision

Supervision refers to activities carried out by health programme or service managers to promote, correct and improve performance. Supervision should not be punitive. Rather, it should be regarded as supportive of staff and their needs for continuing education. Staff supervision examines the performance of individual staff members as well as the output of the entire health care team. On occasion, supervisors may also consult patients and the community to assess staff performance (Flahault et al., 1988). Systematic, supportive supervision and established lines of responsibility and authority will improve the quality of care and enhance staff morale.

Effective supervision should be based on clear service protocols, assignment of tasks to appropriately trained staff, and performance indicators. Supervisors should monitor staff frequently to ensure that protocols are being followed and that the level of competence as reflected in performance indicators is adequate. Some techniques for reviewing job performance are:

- direct observation of staff at work;
- review of case records;
- use of checklists enumerating the key criteria for standard activities (see Annex 3B and C);
- interviewing women about the care they have received.

On the basis of the findings, managers should provide frequent feedback to employees through individual discussion, demonstration of techniques and procedures, periodic staff meetings, and in-service training. Feedback should include both positive reinforcement and specific recommendations for improvement. Ideally, supervisory feedback to staff should include periodic formal written evaluations. The identification of performance problems may indicate the need for changes, such as the use of incentives to improve performance, revision of protocols, or reassignment of tasks.

Supervision is usually an additional task assigned to staff who have a variety of other duties. The role of supervisor must be clearly specified and communicated, and training in the special skills required to supervise staff should be made available.

Supervision in an abortion care setting is not significantly different from that required for other gynaecological and obstetric clinical services. However, supervision of staff who are involved with referral is worthy of a particular note. Regional supervisors must maintain close contact with personnel throughout the referral network in order to ensure competence throughout the system. Regular supervisory visits and frequent communication can improve the quality of care throughout the referral network (see Chapter 11).

Staff attitudes

High quality abortion care is an essential component of all health care services for women. Managers have a responsibility to instil this concept in all staff by setting a positive personal example, providing regular opportunities for in-service training and offering supportive supervision. Managers must create an awareness among staff of the need for psychosocial support of patients and the influence staff attitudes have on the quality of abortion care provided. Whatever the personal perspectives of staff members, managers should ensure that trained staff are available at all times to provide emergency care for abortion complications.

A positive, non-judgemental attitude towards women seeking abortion care is especially important. In facilities that provide elective abortion, it is important that staff understand and support the provision of such services.

Stress can affect staff attitudes and, hence, the quality of service. In a facility with a high caseload of emergency abortion care or one that delivers primarily elective abortion, the staff may experience high levels of stress as a result of focusing exclusively on this emotional issue. Staff, specialists in particular, may resent having to devote large portions of their time to abortion care. In addition to staff rotation, careful supervision, and ample opportunity for discussion, supervisors may wish to consider alternative incentives for staff such as performance awards or public recognition of achievements to help staff cope with the stress. Managers should recognize the effect of stress on their own performance. Two ways to cope with stress that can be helpful for staff at all levels are regular and honest communication about the causes of stress and inclusion of intervals of rest on every shift.

References

ABBATT FR, MEJIA A (1988) *Continuing the education of health workers: a workshop manual.* Geneva, World Health Organization.

FLAHAULT D ET AL. (1988) *The supervision of health personnel at district level.* Geneva, World Health Organization.

Chapter 11

OVERCOMING OBSTACLES TO ACCESS THROUGH DECENTRALIZATION, REFERRAL, TRANSPORT AND COORDINATION

> Many maternal deaths occur at first referral level, either because women come from too far and arrive too late, or because the essential obstetric care they urgently need is not available (WHO, 1991).

To be truly effective in preventing abortion morbidity and mortality, emergency abortion care must be accessible through the existing health care system to all women on a 24-hours-a-day basis. Health care facilities and trained medical providers are usually concentrated in the cities while most of the world's population lives in rural areas, so that women in rural and remote areas are generally either unserved or underserved. For example, 90% of the 200 obstetricians working in Nigeria in 1980 were based in Lagos or state capitals (Armstrong, 1990).

In order to improve the accessibility of abortion care, managers should design health services to include the following:

- provision of care at the lowest level that has the trained staff and appropriate equipment to provide safe care;
- effective referral networks and practices;
- adequate transport between levels of care;
- coordination between units within larger referral facilities.

Delegation of functions between the different levels of abortion care

Delegation of functions between the different levels of care or provision of abortion care at the lowest level possible allows women to obtain care closer to their home. Reducing the time spent in seeking and waiting for abortion care removes a major obstacle faced by many women (Thaddeus & Maine, 1990).

Each level of the health care system has a role to play in the provision of emergency abortion care. If the bulk of this care is

97

shifted to the lowest level feasible, most women can be served promptly, leaving only those requiring the most intensive specialized services to be served by the secondary and tertiary levels.

The primary tasks in managing a decentralized system are to plan for the most appropriate service delivery at each level of the system and to provide an effective referral system for complicated cases on a 24-hours-a-day basis. Clear and specific written protocols or operational plans are needed for the delivery of high-quality services in a decentralized system. In abortion care, protocols should be established and communicated to all staff, covering at least the following issues:

- types of clinical services to be delivered at each level of care, focusing on maintaining service delivery at the lowest appropriate level (see Chapter 2);
- clinical guidelines on emergency abortion care, including specific indications for referral (see Chapter 5);
- channels of referral, i.e., staff at each service point must know to what centre(s) they may refer patients (see below);
- communication of medical information on all patients referred (see below);
- transportation mechanisms for patients referred (see page 99).

These protocols must be clearly stated, accepted and used at all levels of the system. They should form the basis of staff supervision and overall programme monitoring. Furthermore, they should be reviewed regularly to ensure continued applicability. It is the responsibility of the manager of each facility to see that providers fully understand service delivery protocols and work with staff to integrate the protocols into their regular working habits.

Referral systems

A carefully constructed and smoothly operating hierarchy of levels of care is the key to reducing morbidity and mortality in abortion care. While the majority of abortion care activities can be provided at lower levels in any health system, the most severe complications require ready access to prearranged referral sites. Prompt communication, decision-making, and transfer of patient information between the units involved are important elements of any referral system.

Indications for referral should be clearly stated in written service protocols and should be reviewed regularly to ensure that they remain relevant. Referral arrangements for each level of care should be communicated to all relevant staff and implemented as required.

Managers should review the capabilities and quality of care in all facilities in the referral network on a regular basis. Since patients generally live in the community where the referring service site is located, any problems or complaints regarding the referral site will probably be brought first to the attention of the local service manager. When a patient is referred, her satisfaction with the services received at the referral site affects her assessment of the quality of services at the referring facility. Open communication between managers of referring and referral service sites can be an important step in resolving any problems that arise. A system of confirmation of referrals should be established to permit effective monitoring of care. In regularly reviewing the referral system, the local manager should focus on:

- clinical outcome of referred cases;
- promptness and efficiency of referrals;
- preparation and stabilization of patients prior to referral;
- transportation arrangements;
- medical follow-up by appropriate levels, as required;
- written communication from the referring facility to the referral centre, preferably using a standard form;
- written communication of patient status and outcome from the referral centre back to the referring facility, preferably using a standard form;
- adherence to protocols for selection of patients to be referred and relevance of these protocols.

Transportation issues

Life-threatening haemorrhage, shock, and surgical emergencies can occur anywhere and immediate transport can save many women's lives, particularly those who have serious complications and those who live in remote areas. In small units without a full-time ambulance service, emergency transfer will require ingenuity and planning. It is important for managers to consider all locally available means of transportation. Community resources for transportation may include: police, military, agricultural extension services, governmental institutions, civil protection organizations, local nongovernmental organizations such as churches and missions, and individual residents.

All available local communication channels can be used to call
for transportation to transfer women to referral facilities (Herz
& Measham, 1987). Community resources such as short-wave
radios or telephones can support communication channels
available in the facility. When services outside the health system
are included in transportation protocols, standing agreements
for the use of these services should be arranged by the
programme manager to ensure that time is not lost in making
arrangements when emergencies arise. These protocols and
agreements should be periodically evaluated and updated by
managers. Any changes should be communicated to all staff to
avoid unexpected difficulties during emergency situations.

Coordination within facilities

Coordination of the services provided within a single facility is
an important issue in improving abortion care. It is the
responsibility of facility managers to see that links between units
providing different elements of abortion care function smoothly.
Unless units are well coordinated, many women will not receive
the care they need even if official protocols specify appropriate
and complete care. For example, a woman with an incomplete
abortion may be treated in the casualty ward but never receive
family planning services, unless either those services are made
available in the casualty ward or referrals to a family planning
clinic are routinely made.

Managers of some first referral, secondary and tertiary care
centres, in particular, must consider the units within the hospital
involved in abortion care and review the linkages and communication among them. Units that need to be coordinated may
include:

- casualty ward;
- obstetrics, gynaecology and nursing departments;
- operating theatre;
- family planning clinic;
- outpatient clinics;
- social work unit;
- central equipment sterilization services;
- pharmacy and equipment supply units;
- medical records unit;
- central laboratory.

Inadequate communication and linkages at individual service points can restrict access to high-quality services.

References

ARMSTRONG S (1990) Labour of death. *New scientist*, **27**: 50–55, 31 March.

HERZ B, MEASHAM A (1987) *The Safe Motherhood Initiative: proposal for action.* Washington, DC, World Bank (Discussion Paper No. 9).

THADDEUS S, MAINE D (1990) *Too far to walk: maternal mortality in context.* New York, Columbia University Center for Population and Family Health.

WHO (1991) *Essential elements of obstetric care at first referral level.* Geneva, World Health Organization.

Chapter 12

QUALITY OF CARE, MONITORING AND EVALUATION

The goal of high-quality abortion care is not simply that services be available, but that the largest possible number of women are able to benefit from quality care. Meeting this objective requires that services be effectively and appropriately managed and that women understand how to obtain them (IPAS, 1991).

Abortion presents an emotional situation for every woman. In particular, unsafe abortions are often accompanied by life-threatening complications and adverse long-term consequences. Therefore, every woman seeking abortion care must be provided with the highest possible quality of care. Achieving this requires a systematic approach to quality assurance at all levels of care. This is a major responsibility of managers.

Quality of care

Quality of care refers to the overall effectiveness and appropriateness of health care. While it is difficult to define and measure quality precisely, a framework of fundamental elements in the quality of care has been developed by the Population Council and is generally accepted in the area of family planning and reproductive health care (Bruce, 1989). Adapted for abortion care, the pertinent elements and questions or issues related to each include the following.

- *Organization of service delivery.* What is the context in which abortion care is delivered? Is abortion care integrated into existing health care services for women? What additional services such as family planning or treatment of sexually transmitted diseases are available at the same service sites as abortion care? Is care available at the lowest appropriate level of the system?

- *Availability of equipment and drugs.* Is logistic support adequate to ensure a continued supply of drugs and functioning equipment? (See page 84.) Are all essential commodities available? Is the most appropriate technology used?

- *Technical competence.* Are all members of the health care team appropriately trained and do they provide care according to relevant protocols? The existence of a quality assurance programme makes an important contribution to technical competence (see page 106).

- *Information given to women.* Do women receive adequate information about treatment, discharge, child spacing and the dangers of unsafe abortion? Do staff provide opportunities for patients to ask questions and understand the responses? (See Chapter 8.)

- *Interpersonal relations.* Do women feel that they are treated in a non-judgemental fashion, with support and respect, in their interactions with staff?

- *Response to patients' concerns.* Do women have adequate opportunity to express their views and does a mechanism exist to respond to any concerns expressed?

- *Choice.* Is a wide array of family planning methods available to enable women who want to avoid or delay pregnancy to make a free and informed choice of method? (See page 60.)

Quality cannot be imposed by the manager; ensuring quality must be part of the day-to-day activities of the entire service. The manager's role is to create an environment in which communication and feedback are encouraged and used to improve the care delivered. A "quality-of-care committee", with representatives of staff, patients and the community, is one way to translate this spirit into action. Each management team should devise its own approach to this issue.

The use of monitoring and evaluation systems is one way to ensure that abortion care is of the highest possible quality. Monitoring informs the management team about ongoing activities and care being provided. Evaluation, on the other hand, assesses and measures the quality of services and the impact of efforts to achieve long-term objectives, such as reducing maternal mortality and morbidity. The documentation and systems described below are necessary tools in the quality assurance process.

Other elements of quality of care, including counselling, interpersonal relations, ensuring access to care, and using the most appropriate technologies, have been discussed in previous chapters.

Monitoring

Monitoring is the ongoing process of measuring how activities are being implemented and their results in terms of output. For managers of abortion care services, this means looking regularly at specific indicators of the quality of care, identifying changes or problems that occur, providing feedback to staff, and intervening to correct any problems identified.

Monitoring can pick up many issues, including a need for in-service training or a change in staffing (see Chapter 10), or a major flaw in the delivery system that requires attention. There are several ways in which activities can be monitored, including: direct observation of staff at work; use of checklists, for example, to evaluate counselling or clinical skills (see Annex 3, parts B and C); examination of clinic records; and discussions with patients, staff and the community. Assessment of the ability and appropriateness of staff is central to maintenance of high-quality care. Assessing staff performance is a continuous supervisory task, as well as part of evaluation and monitoring. Checklists of critical skills based on current protocols and job descriptions are very effective and objective tools for assessing performance.

Evaluation

Evaluation refers to the measurement of progress towards meeting the objectives of a programme or activity. In abortion care, indicators should be established regarding the efficiency and impact of activities leading to reduced maternal mortality and morbidity. While monitoring looks at the day-to-day implementation of services and is continuous, evaluation refers to a periodic review of the impact of a change that has been introduced. For evaluation to be meaningful, it must be focused on indicators of achievement of objectives that can be measured and verified. Evaluation is not an end in itself, but should be used to identify changes needed and thus lead to improved services within an overall quality assurance process.

As part of the programme planning process, project managers should always consider how a programme will be evaluated, matching the evaluation strategy to the programme's objectives. For example, in a programme designed to decentralize comprehensive abortion care services, an evaluation strategy should be integrated into the plans from the beginning as in the example shown in Table 13.

Table 13. Example of evaluation strategies for an abortion care service decentralized to the primary level

Programme objectives	Evaluation strategies
1. To offer emergency abortion care at all primary health care centres and refer patients according to a specified referral scheme.	● Review primary level service reports and records to determine whether all centres have provided emergency abortion care. ● Review records to determine whether treatment and referral protocols are properly followed for a specified percentage of patients. ● Interview women to assess whether they received prompt local treatment or referral.
2. To ensure that all women treated for abortion receive family planning counselling and receive the services they desire.	● Review records to determine whether all abortion patients have received counselling and desired services. ● Observe staff and patient interactions on family planning by following a number of patients through the process. ● Interview women to see whether they understand the information they have received and whether they received the desired services.

Record-keeping

Accurate and well organized records are essential for monitoring and evaluation as well as for patient care and quality assurance. An organized system of standard concise records facilitates service delivery and provides data for management. Records are particularly important in emergency abortion care services.

A management information system is an essential tool for monitoring and evaluating services; by definition, it is a means of collecting information on the care of patients and using it in service management. For example, information on abortion care that may be reported to the management team at each service site on a regular basis includes:

● the number of women attending the service site by type of care provided;

● the number and category of staff;

● the number and type of services provided;

● the number of referrals and the reasons;

- occurrence of clinical complications as established by service protocols;
- the number and type of critical events related to clinic operations (for example, an ambulance that did not run when needed causing a delay in transporting a patient for emergency care);
- supplies used.

While separate patient record files may be kept in some programmes, many facilities use a logbook to collect essential service data. Annex 4A gives an example of a page from a daily logbook for uterine evacuation procedures, which may be adapted as required. If the most important aspects of care are included in a carefully maintained logbook and the data are summarized regularly, the resulting information can provide an accurate measure of the quantity and the appropriateness of care delivered. In addition, the management team should conduct a periodic review of patient waiting time and duration of stay, since these have been demonstrated to be important indicators of patient satisfaction.

The most useful management information systems are simple and streamlined to collect only the information that is essential and will be used. A complex system that collects too much information is difficult to maintain and to use.

Ensuring the medical quality of abortion care

Managers must determine whether clinical abortion care services meet a minimum standard of medical safety, based on established norms. In doing so, the following sequence of activities could be followed:

- Review current norms and practice.
- Set standards.
- Regularly compare practice with standards.
- Assess results.
- Modify and improve the programme according to what has been learned.

Clinic managers should examine the medical records for indicators of provider skills, such as the number of re-evacuations needed, the number of referrals made and the reasons for referral, and complications and deaths associated with abortion care. This requires accurate and complete record-keeping, periodic review of history forms, observation and analysis. Managers should be responsible for ensuring that the clinical staff hold regular meetings and give feedback on quality assurance. Service statistics, areas of concern, causes of problems (administrative, logistic or service quality), extent and cause of morbidity and mortality, and how to prevent recurrences of adverse events should be discussed at these meetings. When giving feedback to the staff, managers should ensure that the purpose of such reviews is not punitive, but rather to improve the quality of services and identify the possible need for refresher training or other remedial action.

Similar reviews of the quality and content of nursing, counselling, and family planning service delivery records, using selected quantifiable indicators of high-quality care, are also useful tools for quality assurance. Such indicators might include postoperative monitoring of vital signs and the percentage of women receiving postoperative follow-up instructions.

In addition to regular reviews, special incident reports should be made for complications such as failed procedures, excessive bleeding, injuries incurred in abortion procedures, operative or anaesthetic complications, or any unusual conditions encountered. These may be entered in an incident book or on a special form (see Annex 4B for an example of such a form which is suitable for adaptation). The clinical supervisor should review the incident book or forms on a regular basis, to determine whether appropriate action was taken, and should discuss them with the staff. The incident book can be used to plan follow-up of adverse outcomes and to retrieve follow-up information from referral units. Unresolved complications should be monitored closely. Any complication is potentially serious and must be dealt with promptly.

Operations research

Operations research is useful for designing and testing interventions to improve the provision and management of abortion care services. Examples of operations research questions in the area of abortion care are:

- What aspects of care are most stressful to the women receiving treatment and how could these be modified?

- What are the unmet needs most often expressed by women and how might they be met?

- How can postabortion family planning service delivery be improved to meet women's needs more closely?

- Can services be provided by nurses or other health care workers rather than by doctors?

- What is the best staffing pattern to ensure rapid, high-quality care for patients?

- Which is the most cost-effective location within a hospital for providing emergency abortion care?

Several publications on operations research are cited in the additional reading list below.

References

BRUCE J (1989) *Fundamental elements of the quality of care: a simple framework*. New York, Population Council.

IPAS (1991) *Strategy for the next decade*. Carrboro, NC, International Projects Assistance Services.

Additional reading

Publications on operations research

BLUMENFELD SN. *Operations research methods: a general approach in primary health care*. Bethesda, MD, Center for Human Services, 1985 (PRICOR Monograph Series: Methods Paper No. 1).

FISHER A ET AL. *Handbook for family planning operations research design*. New York, Population Council, 1983.

GALLEN M, RINEHART W. Operations research: lessons for policy and programs. *Population reports*, 1986, Series J, No. 31.

BATHIJA H. *Experiences in implementing the WHO protocol for estimating the cost to health services*. New York, Population Council, 1989 (Methodological issues in abortion research).

Chapter 13

COST-EFFECTIVE MANAGEMENT OF ABORTION CARE SERVICES

> The decisions a manager makes about how and where emergency abortion care is delivered can have an effect on the overall cost to the health care system. Managers must decide how to allocate resources in order to provide the highest possible quality of care at the lowest possible cost throughout the system.

In countries with a large emergency abortion caseload, the provision of curative care consumes an inordinate share of scarce health care resources. Hospitalization for treatment of abortion complications taxes already overburdened health resources out of proportion to the actual number of women served in terms of requirements for hospital beds, blood transfusions, medicine, and personnel (Khan et al., 1984; Germain, 1987). Treatment of women with infections places the greatest demand on a hospital's resources; women with sepsis or infection are much more likely to have had an unsafe induced abortion than a spontaneous abortion (Fortney, 1981). Many studies document that up to half of all hospital obstetrics and gynaecology beds in certain countries are dedicated to treatment of women with complications of unsafely performed abortions, and up 50% of maternity hospital resources are used to treat these patients. Conversely, studies of elective abortion generally show that providing this service leads to savings in money and other scarce resources otherwise required to treat the complications of unsafe abortion. (See Liskin, 1980 and Royston & Armstrong, 1989 for reviews of comparative cost studies.)

Abortion care costs can be assessed from many different perspectives. For example, the cost of emergency abortion care can be compared with the cost of performing abortion as a safe, elective procedure; or the cost of treating complications from unsafe, induced abortion can be compared with the cost of preventing unwanted pregnancy. Further, the proportion of total health care costs spent on emergency abortion care services, either nationally or locally, can be determined. Nearly all studies on any of these comparisons have concluded that the provision of emergency abortion care is an expensive service and a drain on medical resources, especially in countries with scant funding for health (Johnson et al., 1993).

Preventive efforts, such as introducing family planning services, have been shown to be effective in reducing the costs of maternal and infant care services, including treatment of incomplete abortion. A study by the Social Security System in Mexico demonstrated that for every peso spent on family planning services, the agency saved nine pesos through reductions in costs for maternal and infant care services. The cost savings included decreases in expenditures for prenatal and postnatal care, treatment of incomplete abortions and infant health care (Nortman et al., 1986).

Budgeting for abortion care

Budgeting decisions depend greatly on local conditions and on programme and medical decisions regarding the care to be provided. The factors influencing cost and considerations related to each include the following.

- *Location of service delivery site.* Costs are affected by the decision to locate services in an outpatient or inpatient setting; to use operating theatres or treatment rooms; to provide integrated or free-standing services.

- *Staffing pattern.* Provision of care by non-specialized physicians or auxiliary health care workers who have been trained is usually more cost-effective because of the shorter and less expensive pre-service training and lower salaries of these categories of workers than of specialists.

- *Medical techniques.* Use of the simplest possible procedures, and those known to have the lowest complication rates and shortest recovery time, reduces the overall cost of care.

- *Ancillary services.* The requirements for ancillary services also influence costs. For example, the routine use of general anaesthesia or excessive testing adds to costs.

- *Caseload.* The total volume of patients and the number of patients with complications influence total costs.

- *Level of care.* Delivery of care at the lowest feasible level with arrangements for effective referral of complicated cases is generally least expensive from a number of perspectives, including transportation, use of specialists, and women's time.

As part of the budget planning process, the responsible manager should consult with medical, supervisory and other knowledgeable staff to determine the costs of abortion care, and how they compare with alternative medical techniques and protocols. Table 14 lists some of the relative cost considerations that might be reviewed for budget planning in order to reduce overall costs.

Budgets include capital (non-recurring) costs and recurring costs (the costs of goods and services that will be paid regularly). Some of the typical categories of capital and recurring costs in health services are noted in Table 15. All of these cost categories should be considered and carefully calculated taking into account information about demand for services or potential caseload.

The cost of providing services may need to be calculated on a per-case basis, broken down into components. Calculations of the cost of the various components of care must be made as accurately as possible in order to facilitate financial planning. Calculations should include *direct costs* or those costs traceable to particular cases and *indirect costs,* which are the general facility costs. Direct and indirect costs of services include the following components:

Direct costs for abortion care

● Disposable supplies used for each case.

● Staff time spent on direct care prorated on a per-case basis.

● Equipment and furnishings used, prorated on a per-case basis over the projected life of each item.

● Transportation, if needed for referral of patients.

Table 14. Relative costs of components of abortion care services

Usually less costly	Usually more costly
Integrated, multipurpose services	Vertical, free-standing services
Trained auxiliary health care workers or nonspecialist doctors	Specialized medical staff, physicians
Outpatient services	Inpatient services
Local anaesthesia	General anaesthesia
Nondisposable supplies (e.g., reusable, drapes, gloves, syringes)	Disposable supplies (e.g., paper drapes, disposable gloves)
Locally manufactured equipment and supplies	Imported equipment and supplies

---

Table 15. Cost categories for health budget planning: capital and recurring costs

---

Capital or non-recurring costs[a]

    Premises[b]
    Personnel training and orientation[c]
    Equipment and non-expendable supplies (e.g., instruments, linen)
    Vehicles for emergency transportation and supervisory visits
    Development of forms and information materials
    Community orientation activities
    Surveys and special studies

Recurring costs

    Premises[b]
    In-service training[c]
    Personnel compensation and benefits
    Pharmaceutical and expendable clinical and laboratory supplies
    Support services (cleaning, laundry, laboratory testing, book-keeping, banking and other clerical tasks, and audit)
    Supervision, monitoring and evaluation
    Information and education
    Reprinting of forms and information materials
    Maintenance and taxes for physical plant
    Maintenance and fuel for vehicles
    Utilities (electricity, water)
    Communications (telephone, telex)
    Office supplies

---

[a] In calculating budgets, capital costs are sometimes prorated over their anticipated lifespan.
[b] Premises can represent either a capital cost (if purchased, constructed or renovated) or a recurring cost (if leased).
[c] Initial training and orientation may be considered a capital cost; however, in-service training must be a regular activity thus representing a recurring cost.

Indirect costs for abortion care

- Administrative costs, including salaries of staff not involved in direct care, divided by the total number of cases treated.

- Rent, utilities and other costs of operating services divided by the total number of cases.

Obviously, some service experience is needed before per-case costs can be determined accurately. Costs should be monitored regularly as changes occur in the components of care and in the caseload, and fees adjusted or levels of reimbursement renegotiated accordingly.

Sources of funding for abortion care

Depending on the health system, emergency abortion care is often provided free or at low cost. In no case should a woman be denied these services because of her inability to pay. Mechanisms for financing elective abortion, on the other hand, vary in different countries and health systems. If elective abortion is funded by national or local governmental resources, financing is relatively simple and straightforward. However, government funding is sometimes unreliable since treasuries and health care allocations are subject to shifts in the overall economic status and political changes in a country.

Government or private health insurance may cover elective abortion; however, this source of financing is often unavailable to many women in need if, for example, it is limited to salaried workers and their dependants. Elsewhere, patients are required to pay for their own elective abortions. Some facilities use a fee-for-service system based on a sliding scale, which charges variable fees according to each patient's ability to pay. Patients are sometimes allowed to pay for abortion care in instalments. In many instances, support is available for women unable to pay for services.

Financial management and audit

Managers of abortion care services must attend to financial management and accounting procedures. Effective accounting and audit systems permit managers to monitor costs, stay within budget, and avoid or anticipate potential financial difficulty. Special accounting procedures may be dictated by the government or nongovernmental agencies providing funds. Internal accounting systems must be designed and maintained with provisions to allow both internal and external audits.

The monitoring of expenditures and adherence to budget is an important aspect of a manager's assessment of programme performance. Responsible management of programme finances should include efforts to improve cost efficiency following the considerations presented in Table 14. Furthermore, managers should meet regularly with staff to discuss financial issues and the role staff can play in reducing costs.

References

FORTNEY JA (1981) The use of hospital resources to treat incomplete abortions: examples from Latin America. *Public health reports,* **96**(6): 574–579.

GERMAIN A (1987) *Reproductive health and dignity: choices by Third World women.* Technical background paper prepared for the International Conference on Better Health for Women and Children through Family Planning, Nairobi, Kenya, October 1987. New York, Population Council.

JOHNSON BR ET AL. (1993) Costs and resource utilization for the treatment of incomplete abortion in Kenya and Mexico. *Social science and medicine,* **36**(11): 1443–1453.

KAHN AR ET AL. (1984) Risks and costs of illegally induced abortion in Bangladesh. *Journal of biosocial science,* **16**(1): 89–98.

LISKIN LS (1980) Complications of abortion in developing countries. *Population reports,* Series F, No. 7.

NORTMAN DL ET AL. (1986) A cost-benefit analysis of the Mexico social security administration's family planning program. *Studies in family planning,* **17**(1): 1–6.

ROYSTON E, ARMSTRONG S, eds. (1989) *Preventing maternal deaths.* Geneva, World Health Organization.

Chapter 14

PREVENTION OF UNSAFE ABORTION: A SAFE MOTHERHOOD INTERVENTION

> The critical point, however, is that there are a number of immediate causes that result in the overwhelming majority of maternal deaths. These are obstructed labour, eclampsia, toxaemia, infection, and complications from both spontaneous and induced abortion. The challenge is that there exist low-cost effective and available interventions that can have a major impact on reducing these mortalities and morbidities if these interventions are specifically planned and practised as a priority.

> What is needed now is dedication and action (Mahler, 1987).

Unsafe abortion continues to take a tremendous toll of life and suffering. The impact of the problem is not limited to the lives of women, their families, and the medical community but affects every sector of society. A number of factors force women to rely on unsafe abortion and lead societies to deny women the care they need. In order to address some of these factors, health care workers need to look for ways of informing and communicating with national and local leaders and communities concerning the magnitude, nature, and implications of the problem of unwanted pregnancy and abortion. Finding the solutions to this problem is not just the responsibility of the health care system. Solutions need to be forged by multidisciplinary teams comprised of both the public and private sector, women's groups, nongovernmental organizations, and community groups, working cooperatively towards the common goal of reducing the morbidity and mortality resulting from unsafe abortion.

The basic elements of a multifaceted effort to combat unsafe abortion are:

- Educating the public about the dangers of unsafe abortion, the importance of family planning for prevention of unwanted pregnancy, and the availability of elective abortion as allowed by law.

- Providing acceptable and accessible family planning and counselling services to prevent unwanted pregnancy.

- Promoting the expansion of services for emergency treatment of all abortion complications through a decentralized health delivery system.

- Providing high-quality medical services for termination of pregnancies resulting from contraceptive failure, for medical indications and for other reasons where allowed by law.

Educating the public

Informing the community about reproductive health concerns, including safe motherhood, is an essential part of preventive health care. Health care managers can play a strong role in disseminating such information to the community. In addition, it is important to gain the support of leaders at several levels for initiatives to improve reproductive health care.

The information required by various community groups, and the best ways of transmitting it, are summarized in Table 16. The main way for hospital and clinic managers to reach various groups in the community is through health education programmes within the health system. All health care workers, in their roles both as service providers and as community leaders, need to be familiar with the topics outlined in Table 16 in order to convey this information to the various community groups. Professional meetings, courses, workshops, and journals or newsletters can be used to transmit this information to health care workers. Furthermore, every health facility should have an established system for communicating new information to staff through seminars or meetings held on a regular basis.

The role of family planning in preventing abortion

Contraceptive services have a vitally important role to play in promoting safe motherhood, whether to prevent further unwanted pregnancy following emergency abortion care or an elective abortion, to prevent additional high-risk pregnancies, or for the primary prevention of unwanted pregnancy. Family planning information and services should be made available wherever abortion care is provided and should be a part of primary health care efforts at all levels, including in the community.

All potential family planning clients should be given full information about available methods of contraception and should be allowed to make a personal choice of method. Having a choice of methods has a positive influence on continuation of contraceptive use, thus reducing the risk of unwanted pregnancy.

Table 16. Information for preventing unsafe abortion[a]

Audience	Content	Where and how transmitted
Adolescent and adult women, their partners or guardians	• Signs and symptoms of spontaneous abortion • Where and how contraception can be obtained • Dangers of unsafe abortion • Current legal status of abortion • Where and how abortion care can be obtained	• Health service facilities • Schools and universities • Workplace • Print and electronic media
Policy-makers and officials	• Health impact of unsafe abortion on women and families • Relative costs of providing emergency care and elective abortion compared with pregnancy care and family planning • Need to legislate for funding of comprehensive, high-quality health services for women	• Reports of research in meetings and legislative hearings with findings presented in a readable format • Print and electronic media • Communications to staff of these officials
Traditional and religious leaders	• Importance of educating constituents to prevent unwanted pregnancy • Relative costs to families and the community of maternal morbidity and mortality due to unwanted pregnancy and unsafe abortion • Current legal status of abortion • How to counsel about pregnancy care and availability of family planning	• Formal and informal community and religious meetings • Workshops by health professionals • Print and electronic media
Health care personnel	• Legal status of abortion care • How to convey required information to groups listed above	• Professional meetings, conferences and workshops • Professional publications

[a] Adapted from Thaddeus & Maine, 1990.

Health care managers and health services staff should be thoroughly familiar with all methods and how they are used, their mechanisms of action, their respective benefits and risks, and the management of side-effects. The information should be provided to clients in a simple and non-judgemental manner and supplemented by written materials designed for the target population.

Expanding access to safe, high-quality emergency abortion care

Expanding access to safe, high-quality emergency abortion care is an essential, life-saving component of any safe motherhood programme. It has been demonstrated throughout history and around the world that abortion is a major response by women to unwanted pregnancy. This is not likely to change, even where contraceptive services are readily accessible. Even where contraception is widely available, unwanted pregnancy can be the result of contraceptive failure. Education about the risks and dangers of unsafe abortion is not likely to change the minds of determined women, even if accurate information reaches all the parties noted in Table 16. Also, spontaneous abortion will continue to occur in a certain percentage of early pregnancies. Therefore, health care policy-makers, managers and service providers must be prepared to provide emergency abortion care of the very highest quality possible, within the limits of the law.

A literature review done in connection with the worldwide Safe Motherhood Initiative has delineated the factors that contribute to maternal mortality (Thaddeus & Maine, 1990). These factors all relate to the following three phases of delay in seeking emergency care for obstetric complications, including abortion:

- delay in deciding to seek care;

- delay in reaching the medical facility;

- delay in receiving adequate treatment.

Fig. 7 illustrates the interaction between some of the factors related to delay in seeking care during the three phases listed above.

To a certain extent, the reasons for delayed treatment are social and cultural in nature and largely beyond the control of the health system. However, several important delay factors can be

Fig. 7.   Factors affecting delay in seeking care

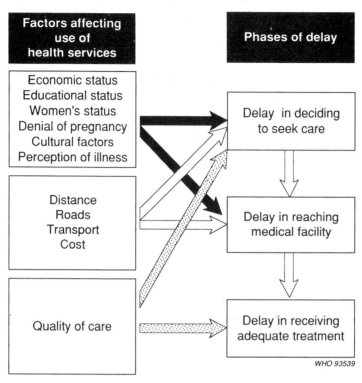

Adapted from Thaddeus & Maine, 1990.

controlled by health care policy-makers and managers. Programme efforts, many of which have been discussed elsewhere
in these guidelines, should be aimed at these factors which
include the following:

- *Increased accessibility.* Managers can improve accessibility by
  ensuring more even distribution of abortion care services,
  maintaining 24-hours-a-day coverage of these services,
  ensuring that referral and transportation mechanisms are in
  place for patients who need to be referred to higher levels of
  care, and expanding training programmes for new categories
  of providers.

- *Increased quality of care.* Managers can improve quality of
  abortion care services by maintaining standards of medical
  quality, providing respectful care, determining and responding
  to women's perspectives, ensuring staff are trained in the
  safest and most appropriate techniques, maintaining essential
  supplies, and giving attention to patient flow.

The role of elective abortion

Providing high-quality medical services for termination of pregnancies resulting from contraceptive failure, for medical indications and for other reasons allowed by law has been shown to lead to a marked fall in maternal deaths. Many of the basic aspects of high-quality emergency care services outlined in the preceding chapters of these guidelines also apply to the provision of elective abortion. It is hoped that, where laws allow elective abortion services, these guidelines will assist managers and policy-makers in service design.

Alliances to improve maternal health

Abortion mortality and morbidity are not just medical issues, they are also social, cultural, and economic issues. Leaders at the local, national and international levels need to recognize the severity of the problem and find solutions through multidisciplinary initiatives that bring together all relevant ministries, cultural and religious groups, and especially women. Policy-makers should lead the fight using all possible channels to focus public attention on abortion mortality. They need to mobilize institutions and individuals in a concentrated effort to upgrade the quality and accessibility of medical care and to change the attitudes in society that contribute to reliance on unsafe abortion practices. If a solution is to be found it must be based on recognition of the fact that protecting women's health is essential to the welfare of a nation as a whole.

Health care leaders and managers must also play a part in this campaign to provide safer and more comprehensive emergency and, where permitted, elective abortion services. The elements of such an initiative in the health care sector include all of the issues discussed in greater detail in the foregoing chapters of these guidelines, which are summarized in the box opposite.

It is only after effective alliances are forged between policy-makers, community leaders and the health care community in support of the prevention of unwanted pregnancy and unsafe abortion—through the provision of better contraceptive services and more comprehensive abortion care—that any impact will be made on the huge maternal mortality and morbidity rates attributable to abortion complications.

Critical components of high-quality abortion care

The safest, most appropriate and most cost-effective abortion care services are those that respond to the needs of the women they serve. The following list presents characteristics of high-quality services:

- Abortion care is available throughout the health care system and each element of care is provided at the lowest level facility appropriately staffed and equipped to provide it safely.

- Care is provided by the least specialized category of health care worker appropriately trained to provide it safely.

- Staff are well trained and well supervised.

- Interactions between the women and the staff are respectful, non-judgemental and non-coercive.

- Women receive counselling and can obtain understandable information on their care.

- Care is provided through outpatient services whenever possible, eliminating routine use of operating theatres and overnight hospitalization.

- Protocols for early referral to higher levels of care as needed and for services to be provided at each level are available and are followed.

- Uterine evacuation is provided using the safest techniques and with the least amount of anaesthesia required to control the women's pain.

- Infection control measures are followed carefully by all staff.

- The family planning needs of all women receiving abortion care are assessed through counselling before discharge, and effective systems for provision of methods, either on-site or through referral, are in place.

- Essential equipment, supplies, and medications are available throughout the health care system.

- Abortion care services are integrated with or linked to the fullest available array of medical or reproductive health services.

- The views of both women and staff are sought in evaluating and adjusting services.

References

MAHLER H (1987) The Safe Motherhood Initiative: a call to action. *Lancet*, **1**(8534): 668–670.

THADDEUS S, MAINE D (1990) *Too far to walk: maternal mortality in context*. New York, Columbia University Center for Population and Family Health.

INFECTION CONTROL PROCEDURES

Adherence to standard infection control procedures in the clinical setting is essential in order to minimize the risk of disease transmission to patients, health care providers or the community. The success of these efforts is dependent on accurately following each step in the chain of procedures that together form an infection control programme.

The infection control procedures described below are intended to supplement measures for routine infection control, such as hand-washing and the use of gloves to prevent gross microbial contamination of hands.

Universal precautions

Since medical history and examination cannot reliably identify all patients infected with human immunodeficiency virus (HIV) or other blood-borne pathogens, appropriate precautions should be used consistently for all patients. Universal precautions (also called universal blood and body-fluid precautions) are recommended for health care workers in all clinical settings to be used with all patients, especially in emergency care settings where the risk of exposure to blood is increased and the infection status of the patient is usually unknown. Universal precautions apply to blood and other body fluids containing visible blood, semen, vaginal secretions and amniotic fluid. The following list of universal precautions is based on practices outlined by the Centers for Disease Control in the USA and the World Health Organization.

- Use of barriers by all health care workers where there is a risk of blood or other body fluids coming into contact with skin or mucous membranes. The type of protective barriers available will vary by health care setting but should be appropriate for the procedures being performed and the potential exposures that may occur.

- Washing of hands and other exposed surfaces with soap and running water immediately and thoroughly if contaminated with blood or other body fluids. Hands should be washed immediately after gloves are removed.

- Precautions to prevent injuries from sharp instruments. Injuries from needles and sharp instruments may pose the greatest risk of HIV transmission in the health care setting. These injuries may occur during procedures, when cleaning used instruments, during disposal of used sharp instruments, and when handling sharp instruments after procedures. Disposable equipment, including syringes, needles, scalpel blades and other sharp equipment, is recommended but is not always available. Used disposable equipment should be placed in puncture-resistant containers placed as close as possible to the area where the equipment is used. Needles should not be bent, removed from disposable syringes, or otherwise manipulated. Recapping of needles should be avoided if possible. Where disposable needles are not available and recapping is practised, the cap should not be held in the hand, but rather placed on a surface, so that the needle can be inserted without the risk of puncturing the skin.

- Steps to minimize the need for mouth-to-mouth resuscitation through the use of ventilation devices.

- Care with skin lesions. Health care workers who have exudative lesions or weeping dermatitis should refrain from all direct patient care and from handling equipment used in patient care until the condition resolves.

Guidelines for sterilization and disinfection of instruments

Sterilization is the safest and most effective method for processing instruments that come into contact with the bloodstream, tissue beneath the skin, or tissues that are normally sterile. When sterilization is either not available or not suitable, high-level disinfection is the only acceptable alternative. High-level disinfection destroys all microorganisms, including hepatitis B virus and HIV, but does not reliably kill bacterial spores.

In order for either sterilization or high-level disinfection procedures to be effective, the instruments should be cleaned prior to processing to remove all organic material. In addition, instruments must be handled properly after the procedures to avoid recontamination.

Sterilization

- Steam sterilization (autoclaving) is preferred for reusable medical instruments including needles and syringes.

Instruments should be sterilized at 121 °C at 1 atmosphere (101 kPa) above atmospheric pressure, for at least 20 minutes for unwrapped items, 30 minutes for wrapped items. Autoclaves must be maintained in good working order and guidelines for time, temperature and pressure settings must be adhered to strictly.

- Sterilization by dry heat is effective for instruments that can withstand high temperatures. It is not suitable for many pieces of plastic equipment, such as syringes. To be effective, instruments must be held at a temperature of 170 °C for 2 hours. A period of $3-3\frac{1}{2}$ hours should be allowed for the entire sterilization process, including heating and cooling. If the maximum achievable temperature is 160 °C, sterilization will require 4 hours once the temperature has been achieved.

- Gas sterilization with ethylene oxide is an effective method. However, use of ethylene oxide gas requires sophisticated facilities and skilled operators, and thus is not widely available in much of the world.

- Chemical sterilization may be considered for plastic equipment that would be destroyed by steam or dry heat. Protocols for the use of chemical sterilants must be followed closely to ensure that the solutions are effective and to protect the patient and the staff from inappropriate exposure. Chemical agents for sterilization include glutaral and formaldehyde.

High-level disinfection

- Boiling in water for 20 minutes is the simplest and most reliable method of high-level disinfection and is acceptable where the equipment required for steam or dry heat sterilization is not available. It is essential that the container used is covered, that timing begins only when the water begins to boil, that all equipment to be disinfected is submerged in the water, and that nothing else is added to the container after the boiling begins.

- Chemical disinfection may be used as a last resort if other means are not available. It is essential that the chemicals for disinfection be used with caution, with meticulous attention to proper protocols for their use. They should be used only if the proper concentration and activity of the chemicals can be ensured. These chemicals can be inactivated by blood and other organic matter. They must be prepared carefully and stored appropriately, away from heat and light, or they may lose their strength and effectiveness.

Note: Many agents are called "disinfectants", but are low-level disinfectants or antiseptics and will not achieve the required high-level disinfection. Among these low-level disinfectants, which should **not** be used for medical equipment are benzalkonium chloride, cetrimide with chlorhexidine gluconate, and phenol (carbolic acid). Care should be taken that appropriate high-level disinfection agents are chosen

Steps in processing equipment for reuse

Equipment used in emergency abortion care that needs to be processed for reuse must be handled carefully to protect both the health care worker and subsequent patients. The following three steps for processing soiled equipment and other items are standard. All three steps must be completed to ensure that equipment is safe to reuse.

- *Decontamination.* Before any equipment is handled, it should be decontaminated by being immersed for 10 minutes in disinfectant solution (e.g. bleach containing 5 g/litre (0.5%) available chlorine) to make the equipment safer for staff to handle. This should be done immediately after the procedure, and it is often convenient to have a plastic bucket containing chlorine solution next to the treatment table. Soiled equipment can then be dropped directly into the solution and allowed to soak for 10 minutes before being removed for cleaning. The solution must be changed daily, or more often if it becomes grossly contaminated, to maintain its effectiveness. Gloves should be worn by all staff handling the equipment.

- *Cleaning.* After decontamination, the equipment should be cleaned and washed well in soapy water. Instruments should be disassembled as needed for cleaning, and organic material should be scrubbed off with brushes (discarded toothbrushes work well). After being cleaned, instruments should be rinsed thoroughly with water to remove any soap residue, which can interfere with chemical disinfection.

- *Sterilization or high-level disinfection.* The equipment should then be sterilized or receive high-level disinfection. The method of sterilization or high-level disinfection chosen will depend upon the characteristics of the equipment and the on-site capabilities. Methods of sterilization and high-level disinfection are described on pages 123–125

Decontamination of environmental surfaces with chlorine-releasing compounds

Wiping with an appropriate intermediate to low-level disinfectant is acceptable for decontamination of surfaces such as table tops.

Most spills of blood in the health care setting should be dealt with by removing visible blood with absorbent material (e.g. paper towelling) and then decontaminating the area by wiping it with an appropriate disinfectant. For large spills of blood or for spills of concentrated or cultured materials (such as may occur in the laboratory setting), the area should first be covered with paper towelling or other absorbent material and then a disinfectant should be poured over the absorbent material and left for 10 minutes. Next, the whole spill should be wiped up with fresh absorbent material and placed in a contaminated-waste container. The surface should then be disinfected with an appropriate intermediate to low-level disinfectant. Gloves should be worn throughout the procedure.

Chlorine-releasing compounds are appropriate disinfectants for the decontamination of environmental surfaces, and sodium hypochlorite is the most widely used compound, e.g. liquid or powdered bleach, eau de Javel. Alcohols are not generally considered suitable for this purpose because of their rapid evaporation and because they quickly coagulate organic residue and do not penetrate it.

Glove use in clinical care

- Use examination gloves for patient care procedures involving contact with mucous membranes.

- Change gloves between patients.

- Use sterile gloves for procedures involving contact with normally sterile areas of the body.

- Ideally, disposable gloves should be used. Do not wash or disinfect gloves for reuse. Washing and disinfecting agents may cause deterioration of the gloves and allow passage of liquid through undetected holes.

- In an emergency situation where disposable gloves are not available, and gloves must be processed for reuse, follow the standard protocols for decontamination, cleaning, and sterilization or high-level disinfection.

- Use gloves when collecting blood samples to reduce the risk of contamination; all blood should be assumed to be potentially infected with bloodborne pathogens.

- Use general-purpose utility gloves for housekeeping chores involving potential contact with blood, such as instrument cleaning and decontamination procedures. Utility gloves may be decontaminated and reused. However, cracked or torn gloves should be discarded.

Waste management

Needles and other sharp instruments or materials should be placed in a puncture-proof container immediately after use and should preferably be incinerated.

Products of conception should be disposed of in accordance with prevailing norms and infection control protocols. Incineration or burial in sealed containers may be appropriate in some circumstances.

Liquid wastes such as bulk blood, suction fluids, excretions and secretions should be carefully poured down a drain connected to an adequately treated sewer system, or disposed of in a pit latrine.

Solid wastes, such as dressings and laboratory and pathology wastes, should be considered as infectious and treated by incineration, burning or autoclaving. Other solid wastes, such as excreta, may be disposed of in a hygienically controlled sanitary landfill or pit latrine.

More information on infection control procedures is available from Maternal and Child Health and Family Planning, World Health Organization, 1211 Geneva 27, Switzerland. Alternatively, managers may contact the following organizations, whose published material was used in the preparation of this annex.

- Centers for Disease Control, US Department of Health and Human Services, Public Health Service, National Institute for Occupational Safety and Health, Atlanta, GA 30333, USA

(Recommendations for prevention of HIV transmission in health-care settings. *Morbidity and mortality weekly report,* **36**(2S): 3S-18S (1987)).

- JHPIEGO Corporation, Brown's Wharf, 1615 Thames Street, Baltimore, MD 21231, USA (*Infection prevention for family planning service programs: a problem-solving reference manual.* Durant, OK, Essential Medical Information Systems, 1992).

- Program for International Training in Health, University of North Carolina, 208 North Columbia Street, Chapel Hill, NC 27514, USA (*Guidelines for clinical procedures in family planning: a reference for trainers,* 2nd ed. rev., 1993).

EQUIPMENT AND DRUGS NEEDED FOR ABORTION CARE

A. Emergency resuscitation materials

Elements of emergency resuscitation	*Materials and equipment*
Management of the airway and respiration	self-inflating bag oropharyngeal airway oxygen supply suction apparatus
Control of bleeding and haemorrhage	oxytocic drugs (ergometrine, oxytocin)
Intravenous fluid replacement	intravenous fluids (intravenous infusion sets)
Control of pain	analgesics, anaesthetics and anaesthetic equipment

B. Essential drugs for emergency abortion care[1]

Primary level

The drugs available at primary level facilities vary from location to location. Nevertheless, the drugs marked with an asterisk in the list given below are useful in expanding the care available at this level. It is important that staff are trained in their use.

Essential drugs for the first referral level

Anaesthetics—general

atropine*
diazepam*

Anaesthetics—local

lidocaine 0.5–2% without epinephrine

---

[1] Adapted from *Essential elements of obstetric care at first referral level*, Geneva, World Health Organization, 1991.

*Analgesics**

acetylsalicylic acid
pethidine (or suitable substitute)

Anti-infectives/antibiotics

broad-spectrum antibiotics:
  ampicillin
  benzylpenicillin
  procaine benzylpenicillin
  chloramphenicol
  metronidazole
  tetracycline
  trimethoprim-sulfamethoxazole

Blood products

dried human plasma

*Intravenous solutions**

water for injection
sodium lactate (Ringer's)
glucose, 5%, 50%
glucose with sodium chloride
potassium chloride
sodium chloride

*Oxytocics**

ergometrine injection
ergometrine tablets
oxytocin injection

Sera and immunoglobulins

anti-D immunoglobulin (human)
tetanus antitoxin
tetanus toxoid

*Skin disinfectants**[1]

ethanol
2-propanol
polyvidone iodine

---

[1] Taken from *Guidelines on sterilization and disinfection methods effective against human immunodeficiency virus (HIV)*, 2nd ed. Geneva, World Health Organization, 1989 (WHO AIDS Series No. 2).

C. Supplies for surgical uterine evacuation

Basic supplies

Intravenous infusion set and fluids (sodium lactate, glucose, saline)
Syringes, 5 ml, 10 ml, 20 ml
Needles:
22-gauge spinal (for paracervical block)
25-gauge standard (for intracervical block)
21-gauge for drug administration
Sterile gloves, sizes 5 to 10
Cotton balls or gauze sponges
Antiseptic solutions: ethanol, 2-propanol, polyvidone iodine or equivalent
Haemostatic chemicals: silver nitrate sticks, Monsel's solution
Long needle holder

Optional supplies for elective abortion

Osmotic dilators, *Laminaria* (small, medium)

D. Instruments and equipment for first-trimester uterine evacuation

Basic uterine evacuation

Tenaculum
Sponge (ring) forceps or uterine packing forceps
Malleable metal sound
Pratt or Denniston dilators: sizes 13 to 27 French
Sharp curette: size 0 or 00
Medium speculum, self-retaining
Container (50-ml) for local anaesthetic
Container (500-ml) for antiseptic solution
Plastic strainer
Clear glass dish for tissue inspection
Long dressing forceps
Container for cleansing solution
Single-tooth tenaculum forceps
Cannulae:
flexible: 5, 6, 7, 8, 9, 10, 12 mm
curved rigid: 7, 8, 9, 10, 11, 12, 14 mm
straight rigid: 7, 8, 9, 10, 11, 12 mm
Silicone lubricant

Vacuum aspiration with electric pump

Basic uterine evacuation instruments plus:

Vacuum pump with extra glass bottles
Connecting tubing

Manual vacuum aspiration

Basic uterine evacuation instruments plus:

Vacuum syringes (single or double valve)
Adapters
Flexible cannulae: sizes 4 to 12 mm

For pregnancy of more than 10 weeks

Basic uterine evacuation instruments plus:

Pratt or Denniston dilators: sizes 29 to 43
Curette: size 1 or 2

Special equipment for dilatation and evacuation procedures

Basic uterine evacuation instruments plus:

Sopher or Bierer forceps

Additional

The following should be available wherever uterine evacuation is performed but not necessarily present on every tray:

Special specula:
    small Pederson type
    large Graves type
    Sims
Uterine sound
Large (sharp) curette
Extra dilator packs
Extra cotton balls or gauze sponges
Needle holder
Tissue forceps

E. Instruments and equipment for second-trimester uterine evacuation

Basic tray for second-trimester abortion

Open-sided vaginal speculum
Atraumatic tenaculum forceps, 25 cm, angled
Pratt dilators, sizes 37/39, 41/43, 45/47
Sponge forceps
Bierer ovum forceps, large, 19-mm jaws
Long dressing forceps
Container for antiseptic solution

Single-tooth tenaculum forceps
1 large and 1 small curette, preferably blunt

Dilatation and evacuation

Instrument tray for instrument storage and tissue collection
Container (50 ml) for local anaesthetic
Container (500 ml) for antiseptic solution
Lidocaine 1% with epinephrine 5 µg (1 : 200 000) in 20-ml
  ampoule
Syringe, 10 ml with control grip for paracervical block through
  25-gauge needle or 22-gauge spinal needle
Gauze sponges
Cotton balls
Vacuum pump, with extra glass bottles
Collection tubing with plastic handle (11-mm inside diameter)
Cannula, uterine evacuation, curved, 14-mm diameter

Intra-amniotic instillation

Instrument tray with sterile cover
Container for antiseptic solution
Dressing forceps
Cotton swabs
Syringe, 10 ml, and hypodermic needle for local anaesthesia
Long needle with a stylet—for instance, a 10-cm 14-gauge needle
  or 18-gauge spinal needle
Syringe, 50 ml
Sterile container for the solution used
Fluids for instillation

Extra-amniotic instillation

Instrument tray with sterile cover
Container for antiseptic solution
Dressing forceps
Cotton swabs
Foley or Nelaton catheter, No. 14 or 18, and a syringe for
  inflating the balloon
Long pincette or forceps for insertion of the catheter
Haemostat for clamping the catheter
Syringe, 50-ml (or smaller, if prostaglandin is used)
Sterile container for the solution used
Fluids for instillation

Equipment for intravenous infusion of oxytocic drugs

Intravenous infusion set, including needles
Intravenous fluids

Additional

The following should be available wherever second-trimester uterine evacuation is performed but not necessarily present on every tray:

Vaginal retractors, 1 pair (medium)
Uterine sound
Sponge forceps, 25 cm, curved
Pratt dilators, full set of largest sizes (to 75)
Needle holder, long
Tissue forceps, 25 cm
Sopher ovum forceps, large, 14-mm jaw
Scissors, large, curved

F. Instruments and supplies for laparotomy[1]

Standard laparotomy set—instruments

Stainless steel instrument tray with cover, 31 cm × 20 cm × 6 cm
Surgeon's gloves—sizes $6\frac{1}{2}$, 7, $7\frac{1}{2}$, 8
Towel clips, Backhaus box lock
Sponge forceps, 22.5 cm
Straight artery forceps, 16 cm
Hysterectomy forceps, straight (Péan), 22.5 cm
Mosquito forceps, 12.5 cm
Tissue forceps, Allis, 19 cm
Uterine tenaculum forceps, 28 cm
Needle holder, straight, Mayo, 17.5 cm
Surgical knife handle, No. 3
Surgical knife handle, No. 4
Surgical knife blades
Triangular-point suture needles, 7.3 cm, size 6
Round-bodied needles No. 12, size 6
Abdominal retractor (Deaver), size 3, 2.5 × 22.5 cm
Abdominal retractor, double-ended (Richardson)
Abdominal retractor, 3-blade, self-retaining (Balfour)
Curved operating scissors, blunt pointed, Mayo, 17 cm
Straight operating scissors, blunt pointed, Mayo, 17 cm
Scissors, straight, 23 cm
Suction tube, 22.5 cm, 23 French gauge
Intestinal clamps, curved, Dry, 22.5 cm
Intestinal clamps, straight, 22.5 cm
Dressing (non-toothed tissue) forceps, 15 cm
Dressing (non-toothed tissue) forceps, 25 cm

---

[1] Adapted from *Essential elements of obstetric care at first referral level*. Geneva, World Health Organization, 1991.

Standard laparotomy set—dressings and linen

Bundles of abdominal swabs with tapes (6 in each bundle)
Vulval pads
Dressing towels
Trolley towels
Abdominal sheets
Mackintoshes, large
Mackintoshes, small
Bundles of radiopaque gauze (6 in each bundle)
Operating gowns, face masks and caps
Plain gauze and cotton-wool swabs
Lithotomy set
Silk sutures in strands (each strand 0.5 m long)

G. Materials for side-ward laboratory tests and blood transfusion[1]

Side-ward laboratory

Test	Materials
Haematocrit (erythrocyte volume fraction)	Microhaematocrit centrifuge
	Scale for reading haematocrit results
	Heparinized capillary tubes, 75 mm × 1.5 mm
	Spirit lamp
	Blood lancet
	Ethanol

Essential materials for the provision of donor blood for transfusion

Blood crossmatching	Patient's serum
	Patient's red cells
	Donor's red cells from pilot bottle
	Sodium chloride solution, 8.5 g/l
	Bovine albumin, 20%
	Water-bath or incubator, 37 °C
	Centrifuge
	Pipettes
	Test-tubes, small and medium

---

[1] Adapted from *Essential elements of obstetric care at first referral level*. Geneva, World Health Organization, 1991.

Collection and storage of blood[1]	Cotton wool and ethanol
	Sphygmomanometer cuff
	Airway needle for collecting blood
	Blood collecting set containing 120 ml of acid-citrate-dextrose solution
	An object for donor to squeeze
	Artery forceps
	Pair of scissors
	Adhesive tapes
	Refrigerator (temperature 4–6 °C) for storage of donor blood. A domestic refrigerator operated either on gas or electricity can be used, but the refrigerator must not be opened too often. A refrigerator that opens at the top is preferable to a cabinet refrigerator.

Sources of emergency gynaecological equipment

Emergency gynaecological equipment is available through international procurement and distribution systems, including the following:

Family Planning International Assistance (FPIA)
810 Seventh Avenue
New York, NY 10019
USA

International Planned Parenthood Federation (IPPF)
Regent's College
Inner Circle
Regent's Park
London, NM1 4NS
England

---

[1] Blood should be collected from healthy adults aged between 18 and 50 years with a haemoglobin level above 11 g/dl. Pregnant women should not donate blood. Individuals can donate blood at six-month intervals.

UNICEF Procurement and Assembly Centre
UNICEF Plads
Freeport
2100 Copenhagen 0
Denmark

United Nations Population Fund (UNFPA)
220 East 42nd Street
New York, NY 10017
USA

Names and addresses of manufacturers and suppliers of
gynaecological equipment are available from International
Projects Assistance Services, 303 East Main Street, PO Box 100,
Carrboro, NC 27510, USA.

TRAINING MATERIALS

A. Training curriculum for vacuum aspiration[1]

This outline presents the most important aspects of training to introduce vacuum aspiration. It is based on courses to train a variety of levels of health care workers in several different countries. The outline should be adapted on the basis of an assessment of the training needs and specific abilities of the participants in the course. If the participants are not already trained and experienced in basic physical and pelvic examination techniques, this content should be added.

Content	*Notes*
Course introduction	The trainer should explain the rationale for holding the course, the learning objectives, and the criteria for successful completion of the course (see Chapter 10).
Pre-test	Where possible, it is advisable to give a pre-test at the beginning of the course. The results of the test should allow the trainers to identify the topics and skills that are needed most by the particular group of trainees.
Maternal mortality and morbidity related to abortion	Trainees should understand the role of abortion in maternal mortality and morbidity in the local setting (see Chapter 1).
Introduction to vacuum aspiration	Trainees should understand the vacuum aspiration technique, including its advantages and disadvantages, indications for its use, limitations, and mechanism of action (see Chapter 6).

---

[1] Adapted from: International Projects Assistance Services, *Vacuum aspiration training curriculum*. Carrboro, NC, 1991.

Postabortion contraception	The lecture or discussion should cover the use of all available contraceptive methods for the postabortion period and explain how to provide methods to women (see Chapter 7).
Equipment	The parts of the aspiration equipment should be identified and the trainer should demonstrate any preparations that the trainees will be responsible for.
Clinical technique	The steps in the aspiration procedure should be explained and discussed. Trainees should then observe a demonstration or an audiovisual presentation of the procedure. If possible, the trainees should perform at least one procedure using a pelvic model before practising in the clinic.
Clinical practice	Trainees should have ample opportunity to develop clinical skills under supervision. The number of procedures that a trainee should complete under supervision will depend on his or her background and training. It is important to allow sufficient time for clinical practice over several days and to set aside time to discuss cases and any difficulties encountered in the clinic. Supervised practice should continue until the trainer is satisfied that the trainee has developed adequate skill. (Section B of this Annex presents a sample form that can be used to evaluate skill in vacuum aspiration.)
Use of medication	The trainer should discuss the use of drugs, including antibiotics, for treatment of infection, analgesia and anaesthesia particularly in relation to shock, paracervical block and uterotonic drugs as required (see Chapters 5 and 7).
Cervical dilatation	It is important for trainees to be able to judge the degree of cervical dilatation and to become skilled in dilatation of the cervix as required for uterine evacuation.

Asepsis	This session should reinforce the need for aseptic technique to minimize the chances of introducing infection.
Diagnosis of complications	This session should cover at least the following: recognition of haemorrhage, sepsis and internal injury (see Chapter 5).
Management of complications	The class should review protocols for management of the complications noted above and discuss cases treated during clinical sessions. Discussion of case studies depicting complications can also be helpful. In addition, ways to minimize intraoperative and postprocedural complications should be discussed.
Infection control	The standard practices of infection control should be reviewed, including the need for use of universal precautions. Infection control practices specific to abortion care should be covered in detail, including decontamination, cleaning, sterilization and disinfection of equipment, and disposal of waste materials (see Chapter 7).
Referral	Participants should be informed of local referral and transport protocols.
Counselling and psychological support	This session should cover the rationale for and importance of thorough discharge instructions and effective interaction with the woman. It should include provision of medical information, family planning counselling, communication of discharge instructions and requirements for informed consent. The class activities should include role-playing. (See Chapters 7 and 8. A sample checklist for evaluating counselling skill is included in part C of this Annex.)
Reporting and record-keeping	It is important to discuss the importance of good record-keeping (see Chapter 12). The participants should practise completing any required forms during training.

Evaluation If training leads to certification it should be dependent on achieving the desired level of skill. Certification should not be given automatically or be based on completion of an arbitrary number of procedures. In order to improve future classes, each course participant should be asked to evaluate the course, giving positive and negative feedback. A confidential survey is very useful for this.

B. Checklist for evaluation and supervision of vacuum aspiration practice[1]

The following checklist is designed to be used during the direct observation of a vacuum aspiration procedure. The evaluator should be experienced in vacuum aspiration. The checklist may be modified and adapted as required.

Part 1. Observe whether the operator adequately:

— Assesses the patient's status (medical history, presenting conditions, date of last menstrual period, and emotional state) and orders necessary laboratory tests.

— Assures that the necessary material, medication and instruments are available in the procedure room before beginning.

— Establishes rapport with the woman, discusses the procedure with her, and is supportive.

— Evaluates the need for anaesthesia, analgesia, or sedation on the basis of the patient's condition and emotional state.

— Assesses the size and position of the uterus, or identifies trauma if present.

— Identifies cervical laceration, dilatation, or trauma if present.

— Administers antibiotics if needed.

— Ensures that the cannulae have been sterilized or disinfected and rinsed free of any caustic solutions used.

---

[1] Adapted from International Projects Assistance Services, *Clinical evaluation form for manual vacuum aspiration*, Carrboro, NC, 1991.

— Prepares the aspiration syringe or pump and checks vacuum tightness.

— Selects the appropriate cannula on the basis of uterine size and cervical dilatation and inspects cannula and syringe for signs of wear.

— Administers paracervical block or other pain control measures, if needed.

— Dilates the cervix if needed without causing trauma.

— Uses no-touch technique; does not contaminate the cannula.

— Moves cannula effectively to empty the uterus.

— Determines when the evacuation is complete.

— Examines the aspirate to ensure that the tissue evacuated is consistent with the patient's condition and history, and sends sample to the pathology laboratory if needed.

— Monitors the patient for complications and treats any that occur.

— Gives appropriate discharge instructions.

— Ensures that family planning counselling is given and provides a method if the woman desires one.

Part 2: Recommendations

If the operator has not yet reached the necessary level of skill, list your recommendations for improving skill, referring to specific items in part 1.

Recommendations

_____

_____

_____

_____

Part 3: Comments

Please add any comments you may have about the trainee's
ability.

_____

_____

_____

C. Checklist for evaluation and supervision of counselling skills[1]

The following checklist is designed to be used for self-evaluation
by the counsellor or in conjunction with observation of
counselling skills by an external evaluator. The external
evaluator should be experienced in counselling techniques. The
checklist may be modified and adapted to conform with the
curriculum used in the original training.

**To assess listening skills, the evaluator should observe whether the
counsellor:**

— Meets clients in a private, comfortable place.

— Accepts clients as they are; treats each one as an individual.

— Listens to what clients say and how they say it; observes tone
of voice, choice of words, facial expressions and gestures.

— Puts himself or herself in the client's place as she talks.

— Keeps silent sometimes, giving the client time to think, ask
questions, and talk.

— Listens carefully to the client, rather than thinking of what
to say next.

— Repeats occasionally what has been heard to ensure
understanding by both parties.

— Sits comfortably, avoids distracting movements and looks
directly at the client.

---

[1] Adapted from Lettenmaier C, Gallen M. Why counselling counts. *Population reports*,
Series J, No. 36 (1987).

To assess questioning skills, the evaluator should observe whether the counsellor:

— Uses a tone of voice that shows interest, concern and friendliness.

— Asks only one question at a time and waits for an answer.

— Asks questions that let the client express her needs.

— Asks open-ended questions that cannot be answered with a simple "yes" or "no", to encourage communication.

— Uses words such as "then?", "and?", "oh?" to encourage the client to keep talking.

— Avoids beginning questions with "why?" since this can connote judgement of the client.

— Asks the same question in different ways to ensure the client has understood a point.

MODEL RECORDS FOR USE IN ABORTION CARE SERVICES

A. Sample page of a logbook for emergency abortion care

Date	Procedure no.	Patient no.	Name of provider	Uterine size in weeks	Analgesic, anaesthetic, sedation: drug and dose	Diagnosis	Procedure				Complications			Discharge instructions given	Family planning counselling given	Contraceptive method delivered if woman desired	Remarks
							Vacuum aspiration	D&C	D&E	Other	Minor	Major	Death				

Key: D&C, dilatation and curettage; D&E, dilatation and evacuation.

B. Example of an incident report form for abortion complications

The attending medical provider should complete this form as soon as possible for all major complications that occur during the provision of abortion care.

1. Patient and procedure

Name:
Date of admission: Time of admission:
Date of procedure: Time of procedure:
Diagnosis:
Type of procedure:

2. Complications encountered

Describe the complication and the time it was recognized.

3. Patient's clinical condition

Describe the patient's condition before the procedure.

Describe the patient's condition after the procedure.

4. Procedure

Describe the details of the procedure.

5. Treatment of complications

Describe actions taken to treat complications and follow-up care required.

_____   _____

Clinician reporting   Location (hospital, clinic)
(print name)

_____   _____

Signature   Date

6. Case review

Appropriateness of care

Treatment required

Follow-up required

Proposed actions to minimize future complications

_____   _____

Supervisor (print name)   Date

_____

Signature